ABOUT THE AUTHORS

Jonathan Barney received his BA degree from California State University, San Marcos. He has over five years' experience as an EMT and Emergency Room Technician. He is currently a fourth-year medical student at the American University of the Caribbean School of Medicine. Following graduation, he intends to pursue a career in emergency medicine.

Dr. Hayden is a career emergency medicine specialist with over 28 years' experience. A graduate of the University of Michigan Medical School, he completed his residency in emergency medicine at Advocate Christ Medical Center, Chicago. He holds a doctorate in education from the University of Memphis.

ACKNOWLEDGMENT

In preparing this manuscript, we extend our sincere appreciation to Dr. Burt Hamrell, Department of Molecular Physiology and Biophysics, University of Vermont College of Medicine, for his review and instructive recommendations.

Copyright © 2018 John Hayden All rights reserved.

The level of knowledge pertaining to electrocardiogram (ECG) interpretation among prehospital healthcare providers undoubtedly affects patient outcomes. Emergency Medical Services (EMS) personnel from Emergency Medical Responders (EMR) to Emergency Medical Technicians (EMT), advanced emergency medical technicians (AEMT) and paramedics play a critical role in the care of acutely ill and injured patients. First responders make critical decisions regarding initial assessment, intervention and transport. They must do so expeditiously. Such decisions have profound implications on quality and continuity of care. The importance of such actions becomes especially evident regarding on-scene ECG interpretation.

A position statement published in 2009 by the National Emergency Medical Services Advisory Council (NEMSAC) states that, "The EMS interventions that have been demonstrated to contribute most significantly to improved outcomes are those that result in earlier diagnosis and more timely reperfusion, specifically the capture and interpretation of 12-lead ECGs, notification of the receiving hospital and activation of coronary care or catheter lab teams, triage directly to a percutaneous coronary intervention (PCI) center, and administration of thrombolytic agents during transport". (*Ann Emerg Me*d. 2011; 57(2):170)

The Heart Disease and Stroke Statistics 2017 report of the American Heart Association (AHA) notes that roughly 790,000 Americans suffer a heart attack every year. A longstanding adage from the AHA that's popular among EMS providers is, "time is muscle", i.e., the shorter the transport time, the more vital muscle can be salvaged in a cardiac emergency such as myocardial infarction (MI).

The AHA recommends a medical contact-to-balloon or door-to-balloon time (D2BT) within 90 minutes, where "balloon" refers to PCI. Therefore, EMS personnel must make decisions expeditiously that decrease both time on-scene and transit time to a facility with PCI capabilities.

Excellent resources for teaching ECG interpretative skills abound on internet as well as in traditional textbooks. However, they do not target first responders primarily. While they contain vast amounts of important detailed information, prioritization as to clinical urgency is not their primary focus. The approach adopted here – **ECG Primary Survey** – provides a simplified clinical method to identify and prioritize life-threatening cardiac emergencies that first responders may encounter. Mastery of the **ECG Primary Survey** also provides a foundation on which to build and expand advanced skills in ECG interpretation.

Using the **ECG Primary Survey approach**, first responders should address these four questions:

1. **Is heart rate too fast or too slow causing cardiovascular instability?**
2. **Is rhythm supraventricular or ventricular?**
3. **Are ST segments consistent with ST-Elevation Myocardial Infarction (STEMI) or NonST-Elevation Myocardial Infarction (NSTEMI)? NSTEMI?**
4. **Are T waves consistent with STEMI / NSTEMI?**

These four questions constitute the ECG "**Primary Survey**", a clinical methodology borrowed from the American College of Surgeons' Advanced Trauma Life Support (ATLS) training manual. ATLS stresses the importance of a "primary survey" to identify potentially life- threatening conditions such as obstructed airway, hypotension, or tension pneumothorax. ATLS instructs caregivers to resolve such lethal issues immediately, taking preference over other interventions. Once Primary Survey issues are resolved, ATLS instructs caregivers to perform a "**secondary survey**", a head-to-toe examination to identify all other non-life- threatening injuries.

In the setting of acute, non-traumatic chest pain in adults, a similar approach seems particularly applicable. The ECG Primary Survey seeks to identity *clinically urgent* cardiac emergencies that are potentially life threatening. As their number one priority, first responders should identify such emergencies and initiate appropriate, immediate, therapeutic interventions within the scope of their care.

A complete 12 lead ECG analysis and interpretation extend beyond elements of the Primary Survey. These include complex cardiac arrhythmias, bundle branch blocks, heart blocks, axis abnormalities, etc. Adopting the ATLS approach, such issues comprise the "**secondary survey**", undertaken once the primary survey has addressed any life-threatening cardiac emergencies due to cardiac rate, ventricular rhythm, STEMI, and NSTEMI. The forthcoming monograph, *Advanced ECG for First Responders*, addresses these "secondary survey" topics.

In myocardial infarction, salvaging cardiac muscle is time dependent. First responders should complete the ECG Primary Survey within minutes. Transmitting radio STEMI or NSTEMI alerts to receiving hospitals will expedite reperfusion strategies. Only repeated practice in recognizing STEMI and NSTEMI on 12 lead ECGs will achieve this proficiency.

The following chest pain scenario serves as your introduction to ECG Primary Survey. The only skill required is your careful observation!

SCENARIO: As a first responder, you are participating in a physician-shadowing experience in the emergency department. The triage nurse has obtained a 12 lead ECG on a 42-year-old man complaining of chest pain. She asks that you show the following tracing to the emergency physician. Examine this ECG carefully before proceeding to the next page.

MR#249076577
Mary Hammons
15:20
2-19-15
Emergency Department

Rate: 75 bpm
Rhythm sinus
P-R 0.16 sec
QRS 0.11 sec
QT 0.38 sec

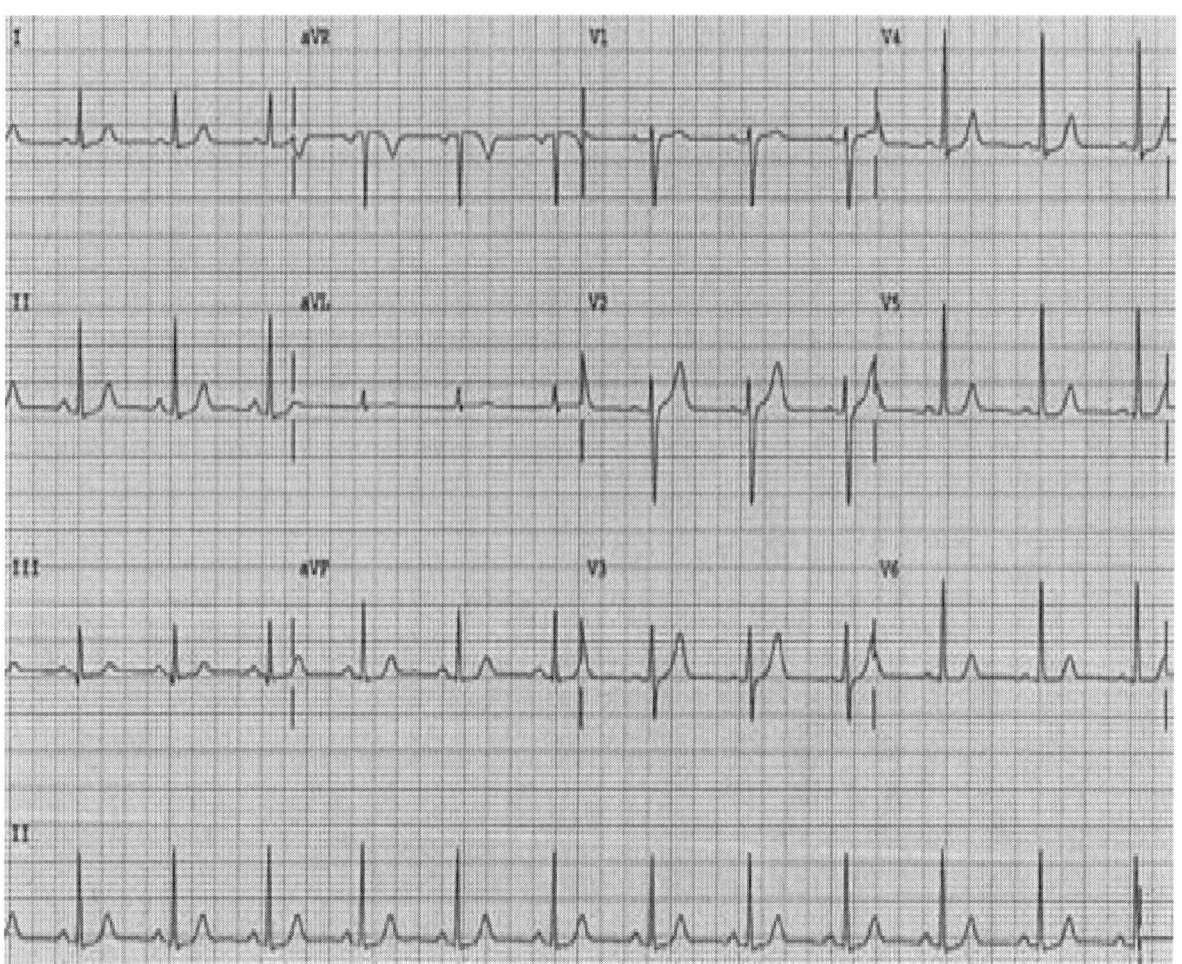

Should you:

Immediately show this ECG to the ED physician or revisit the triage nurse?

Even if you know little or nothing about ECG interpretation, you should be able to answer this question!

ANSWER: Revisit the triage nurse. Why? Because this is not the patient's ECG! Did you look carefully at the patient demographics? This ECG belongs to Mary Hammons – not a 42-year-old male with chest pain.

Mary Hammons

MR#249076577 **Rate: 75 bpm**
Rhythm sinus
15:20   P-R 0.16 sec
2-19-15   QRS 0.11 sec
Emergency Department   QT 0.38 sec

Always make sure you confirm and or document patient identifying data on every ECG you perform! In a busy emergency department, there may be several ECGs awaiting physician review. The same is true in coronary care units, where physicians may repeat ECGs several times a day. To avoid mistaken identity, always include patient identifying data, including date and time. Failure to do so may lead to mistakes in management and treatment.

Checking patient identification is critical not only for ECGs but for other studies, such as x- rays, laboratory test results, and all other patient reports. Do not forget to verify patient's ID bracelets. The initial step in the ECG Primary Survey is to confirm the patient's identifying demographics!

The 12 Lead ECG

Before discussing the Primary Survey, we need to identify the components of a 12 lead ECG. Examine this ECG:

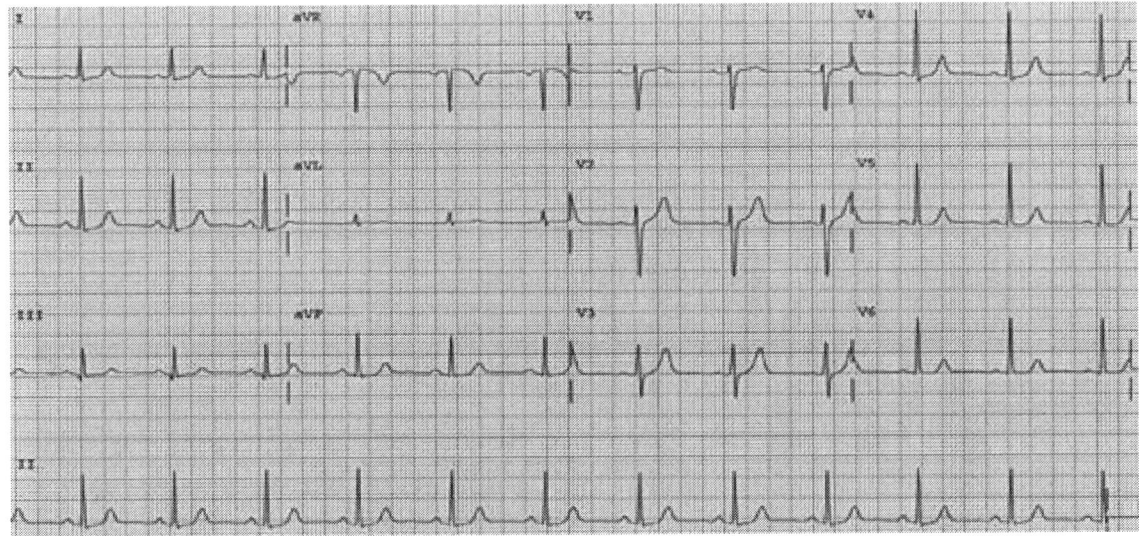

On the same ECG below, we have drawn rectangles to identify the location of each lead. The bottom portion of the ECG contains the rhythm strip, usually Lead II. Note the lead designations in the upper left-hand corner of each rectangle.

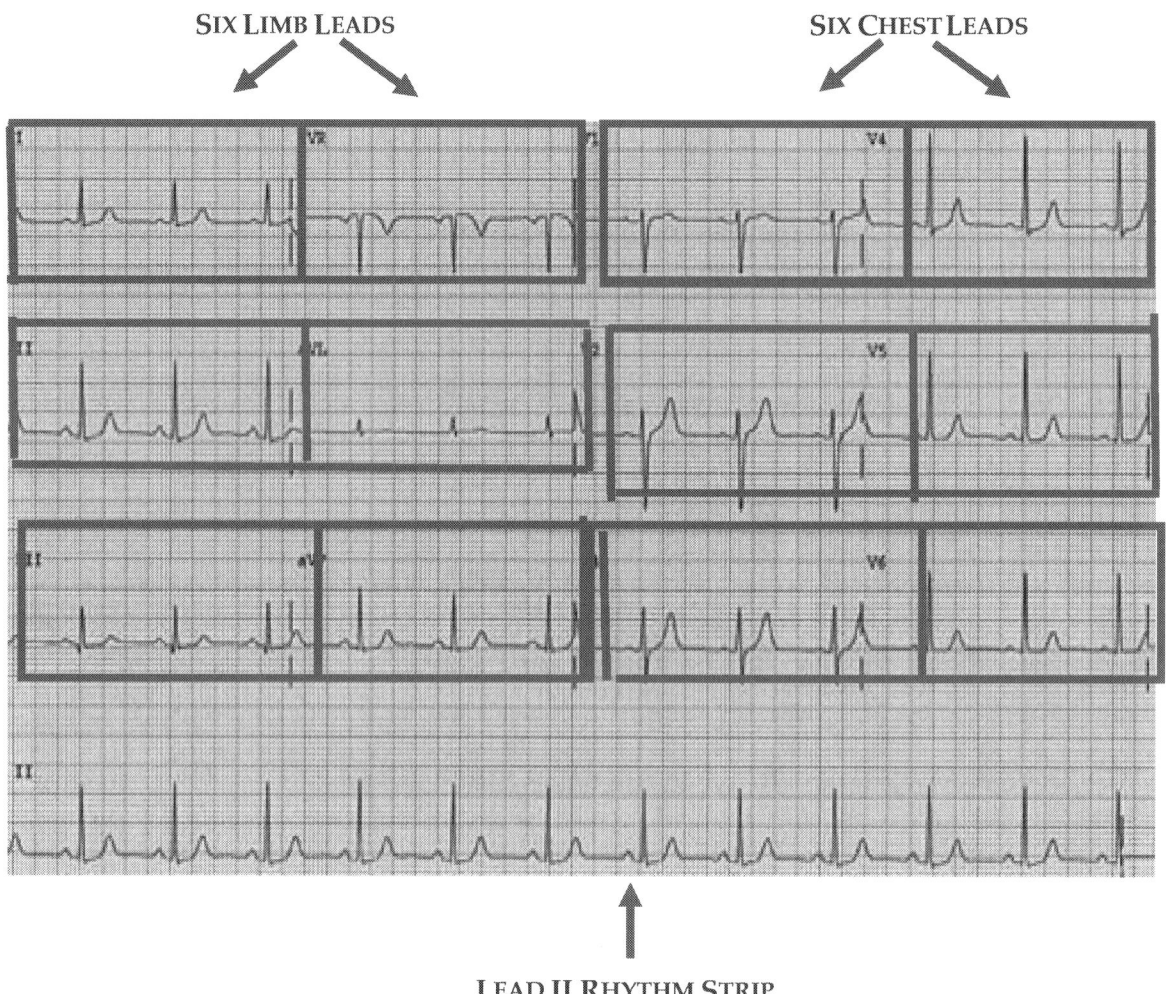

Four skin electrodes positioned on the limbs and six chest electrodes attached to the chest produce the 12 lead ECG. A 12 lead ECG tracing usually contains a rhythm strip as shown, usually Lead II, because that lead more clearly displays *p* waves. Sometimes chest lead V1 or V2 is used for the rhythm strip. A longer rhythm strip is often necessary to detect rhythm abnormalities beyond what appears in a single lead, which is why a longer Lead II rhythm strip appears at the bottom of the tracing.

Notice that in each lead below there are three heartbeats indicated by numbered QRS complexes. A straight-line artifact separates one lead from another. Do not mistake these artifacts as heartbeats. The blue arrows identify these lead dividers.

Heart Beats

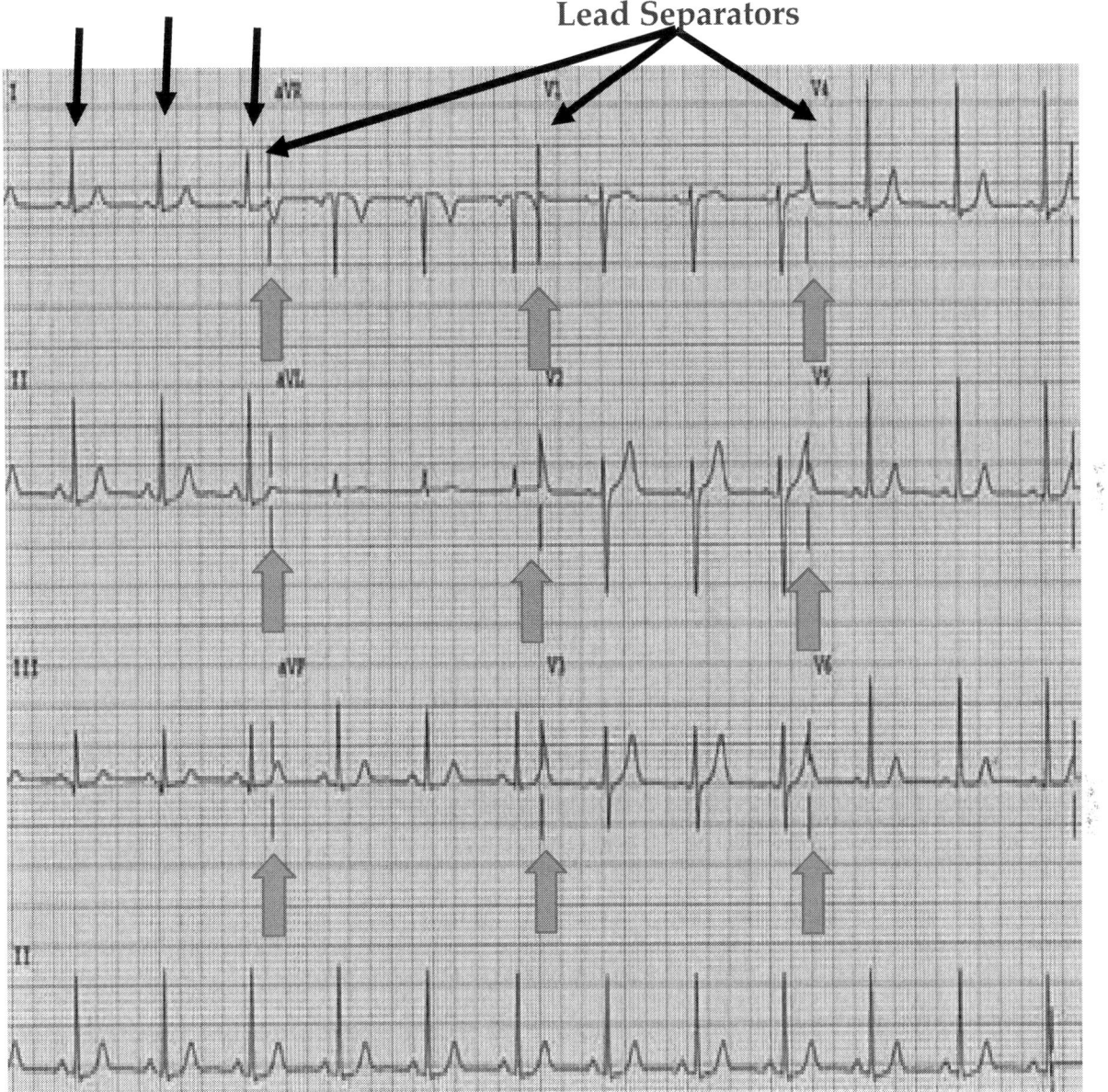

Lead II Rhythm Strip

ECG leads provide critical information about where injury is occurring. Each lead views the heart from a different angle recording electrical activity in various anatomic locations of the heart. As a result, leads can localize areas of ischemia and infarction.

EXERCISE– ECG CASE 1

COMPLETE THIS EXERCISE BEFORE VIEWING THE CASE SOLUTION YOUTUBE VIDEO.

Case 1: Components of the 12 Lead ECG
1. In the following ECG, label each lead.
2. Draw a rectangle around each limb and chest lead.
3. Identify the rhythm strip.

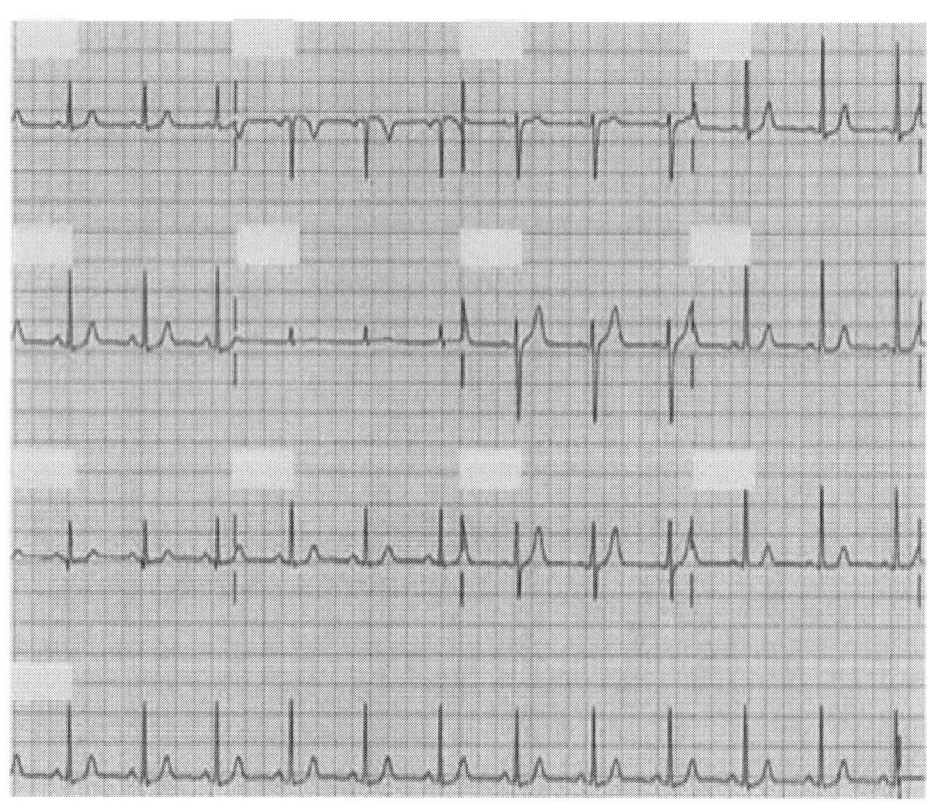

Video Companion link: https://youtu.be/a-fx6BgyIrs

Timestamp 0:00 Beginning

Using ECG Leads to Localize STEMI / NSTEMI

ECG leads can identify where in the heart myocardial ischemia or infarction occurs as well as what coronary artery is involved.

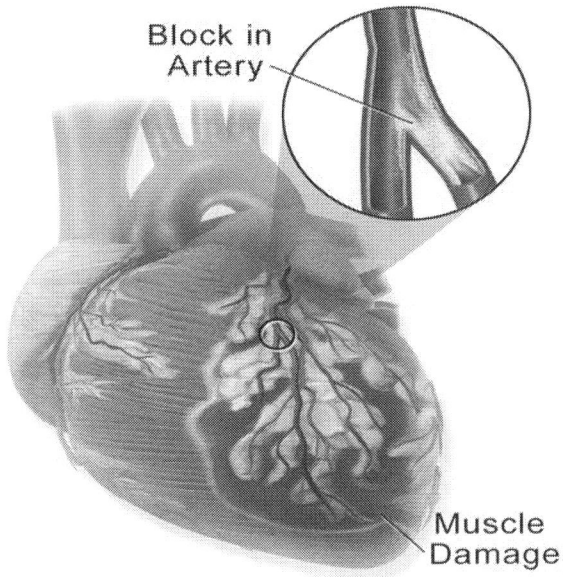

Heart Attack

The 12 lead ECG acts like a camera that produces 12 pictures (leads) of the electrical activity or patterns in specific regions of the heart, primarily the left and right ventricles. Each "picture" has a label, e.g., lead I, lead II, V1, etc. An abnormal pattern such as ischemia or infarction (STEMI) appearing in that lead helps identify the location of injury as well as which coronary artery may be involved.

Skin electrodes applied to the body record the heart's electrical activity. Leads represent imaginary lines between electrodes. A 12 lead ECG produces 12 tracings: six limb leads and six chest leads.

Four limb electrodes are placed on the limbs but alternatively can be placed on the shoulders and hips to reduce ECG interference and artifact. Although only four limb electrodes are used, in effect, they produce **SIX** tracings on the ECG as explained by Einthoven's Triangle: I, II, III, aVL, aVF, aVR.

Einthoven Triangle

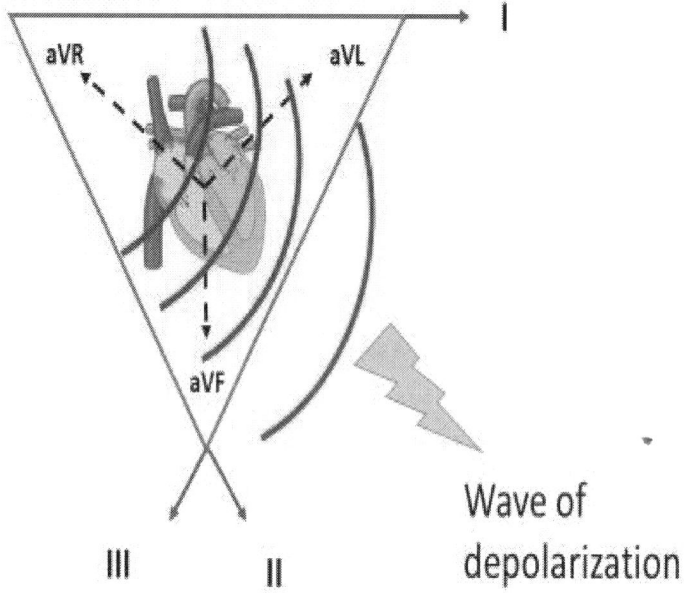

Willem Einthoven (1860-1927) was a Dutch doctor, physiologist who developed the technology for producing clinically useful ECG recordings and understanding of the biophysics. He received the Nobel Prize in Medicine for doing so.

Beginning at the SA node, the wave of depolarization spreads downward diagonally from right to left as pictured. ECG leads viewing the approaching depolarization wave will have upright QRS-T wave complexes (aVL, I, II, aVF, III). The QRS-T wave complex in aVR will normally appear inverted, since that lead sees the depolarization wave moving away. For additional information on Einthoven's Triangle, see

https://en.wikipedia.org/wiki/Einthoven%27s_triangle.

Roman numerals and letters designate limb leads: **I - II - III - aVR** (augmented vector right) - **aVL** (augmented vector left) / **aVF** (augmented vector foot). In addition to limb leads, six skin electrodes are attached to the chest. Four limb leads and six chest leads produce the 12 lead ECG tracing. Augmented vector terminology refers to directional electrical forces at play during the cardiac cycle.

Chest leads are designated V1-V2-V3-V4-V5-V6. The following picture shows placement of chest leads. These leads view the heart in the horizontal plane from front to back.

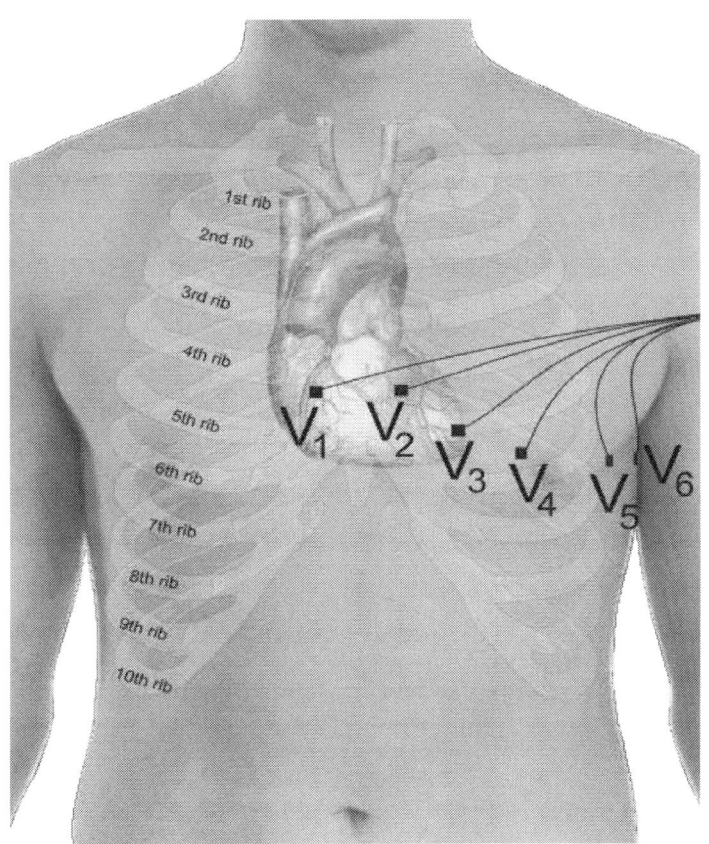

Häggström, M (2014). "Medical gallery of Mikael Häggström 2014". *WikiJournal of Medicine.* Creative Commons. Used with permission.

Keep in mind that this arrangement of skin electrode placement is typical for a standard 12 lead ECG. However, certain clinical situations may warrant repositioning electrodes to evaluate other cardiac abnormalities. For example, when a patient suffers blockage of the right coronary artery and subsequent right ventricular infarction, position chest electrodes on the *right* side of the chest to demonstrate more clearly right ventricular STEMI. To evaluate a posterior wall myocardial infarction that may be easily missed, place electrodes on the back of the chest to reveal characteristic ST segment elevation not seen in anterior chest leads.

For additional information on alternate lead placement, see

https://www.youtube.com/watch?v=ytwu3FLsqtI

Understanding Limb Leads

A simple analogy using satellites and cameras may explain how leads function and what they tell us. The following illustration demonstrates this concept.

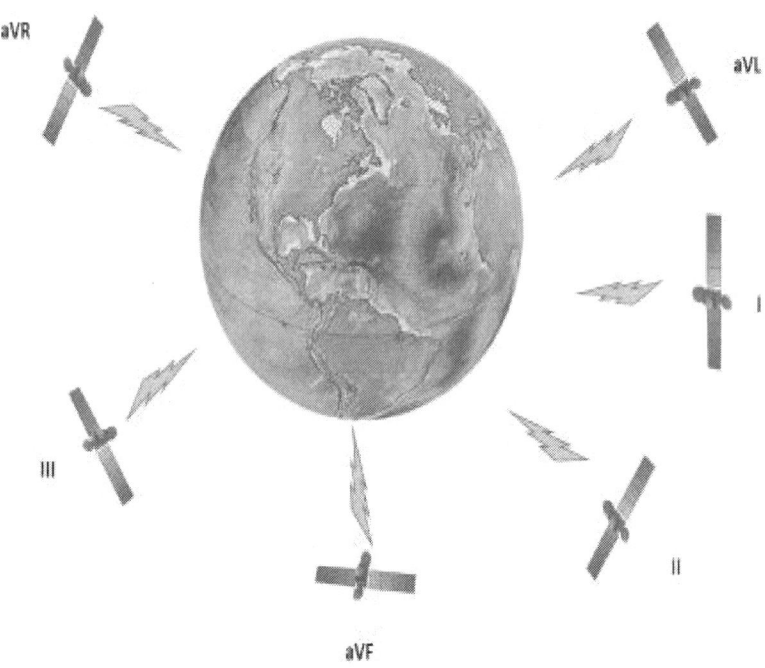

In this picture, six satellites circle the earth, each labeled with ECG designations. Looking at the picture, what part of the earth is satellite aVL viewing?
What about satellite II?

What about the remaining satellites?

Satellite aVL focuses on Africa and satellite II focuses on the Atlantic Ocean. aVF views South America, while aVR focuses on the Pacific Ocean.

Let us replace the earth with a heart and satellites with cameras. Just as satellites circle the earth and record activity in specific geographic regions, limb leads encircle the heart and are poised to record the electrical activity in the anatomic areas on which they focus, thereby producing the typical ECG.

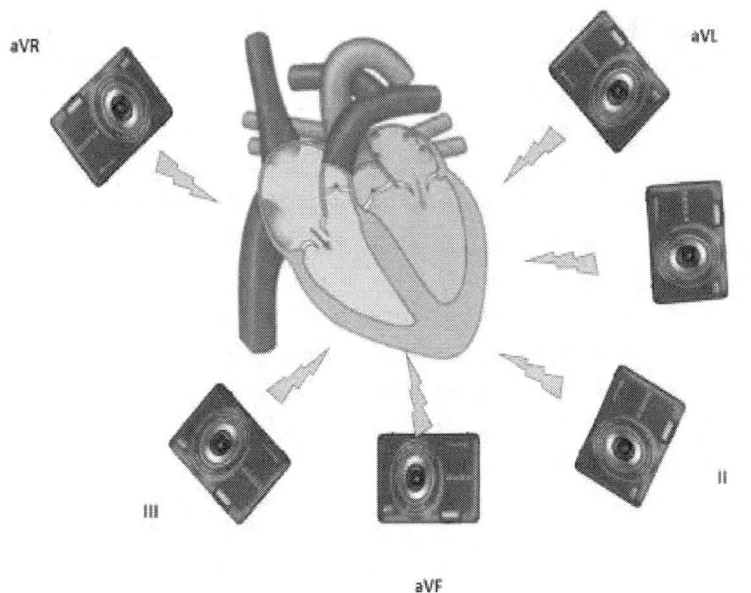

Examine the above cameras (leads). Two "cameras" focus exclusively on the left ventricle: leads aVL and I. Two leads focus exclusively on the right ventricle: leads aVF and III. Lead II focuses on the apex of the heart that includes a portion of BOTH ventricles.

Notice on the 12 lead ECG, the QRS complex in aVR is inverted because the direction of current is down and to the patients left. The wave of depolarization is moving away from aVR, a positive terminal, toward the negative end of the aVR axis.

These limb leads capture the electrical patters occurring in the ventricles. In doing so, they can identify abnormal electrical patterns on the ECG such as those produced by ischemia or infarction.

In the frontal plane, limb leads focus on what is occurring in both ventricles. Why ventricles? Because these are the muscular "pumps" that maintain cardiac output. Leads identify electrical abnormalities such as arrhythmia, ischemia, or infarction that may affect cardiac function. For example, if there is a myocardial infarction affecting the left ventricle, the infarction pattern will appear in those limb leads focused on the left ventricle, namely: Leads I, II, and aVL.

LIMB LEADS FOCUSED ON THE LEFT VENTRICLE

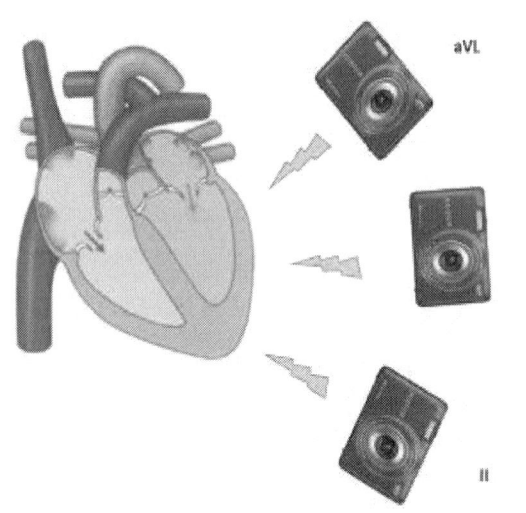

Limb Leads Focused on Left Ventricle I - II - aVL

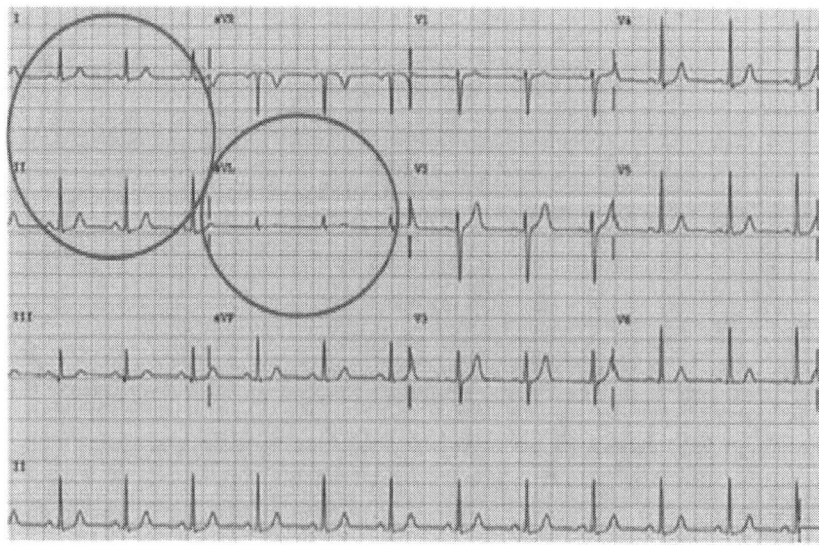

Likewise, if there is a myocardial infarction affecting the right ventricle, the infarction pattern will appear in limb leads II, III, and aVF.

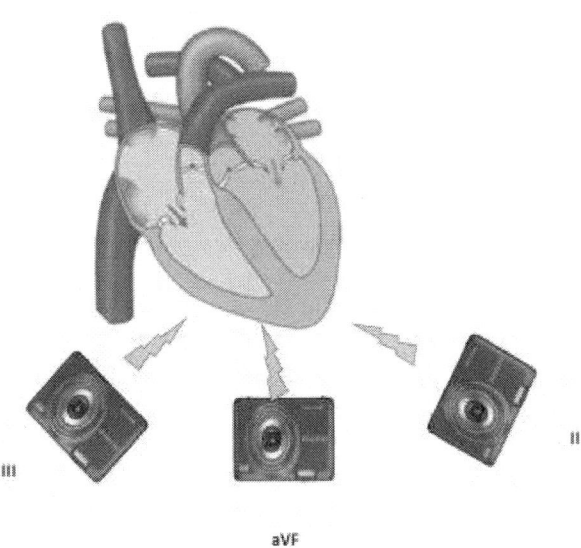

LIMB LEADS FOCUSED ON THE RIGHT VERNICLE

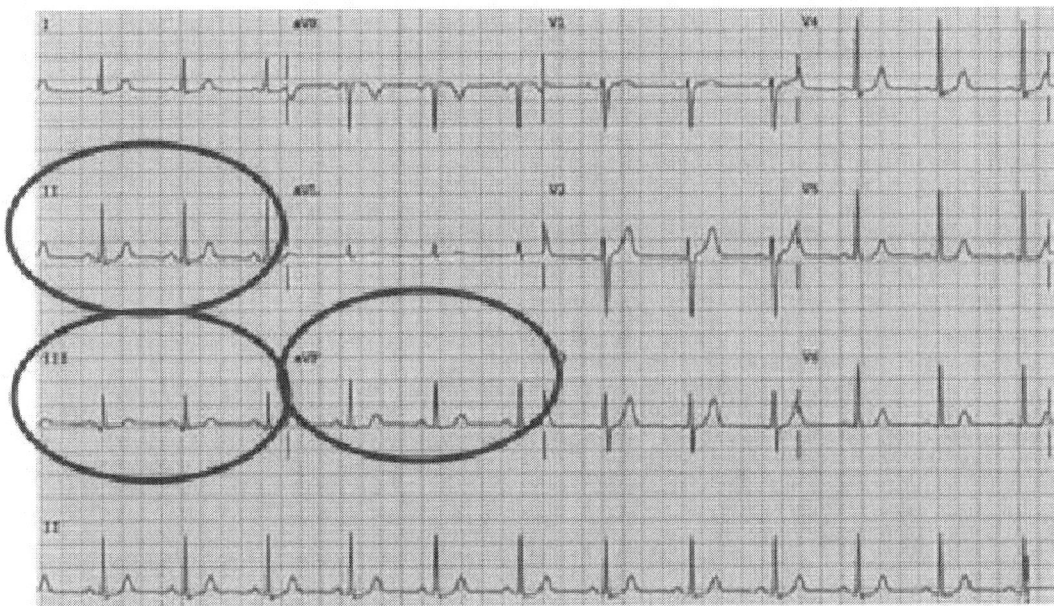

Limb Leads Focused on the Right Ventricle
II –III - aVF

What about limb lead aVR? Some authors have referred to aVR as the "forgotten lead" because it does not focus on either ventricle. However, research suggests that elevated ST segments in this lead signify increased mortality in the setting of acute myocardial infarction. See https://www.medscape.com/viewarticle/589781.

Understanding Chest Leads

Chest leads, also referred to as precordial leads, function in the very same manner as limb leads. However, rather than seeing the heart in a frontal plane, these leads view the heart in cross-sectional plane, i.e., from front to back, as red arrows demonstrate in the following picture.

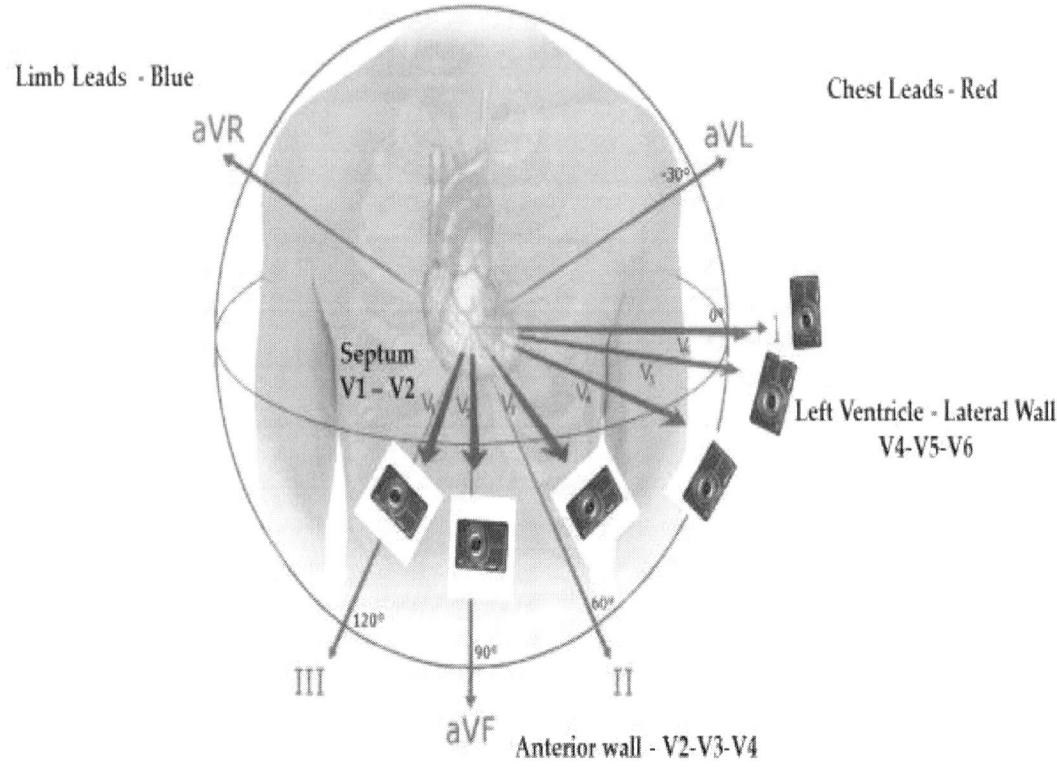

2015-03-17 05 Npatchett, MD
Modified from Wikimedia Commons

Chest lead "cameras" focus on three specific areas of the heart, namely, the septum (V1-V2), the anterior wall of the left ventricle (V2-V3-V4), and the lateral wall of left ventricle (V4-V5-V6).

Chest leads V1-V2 view the septum.

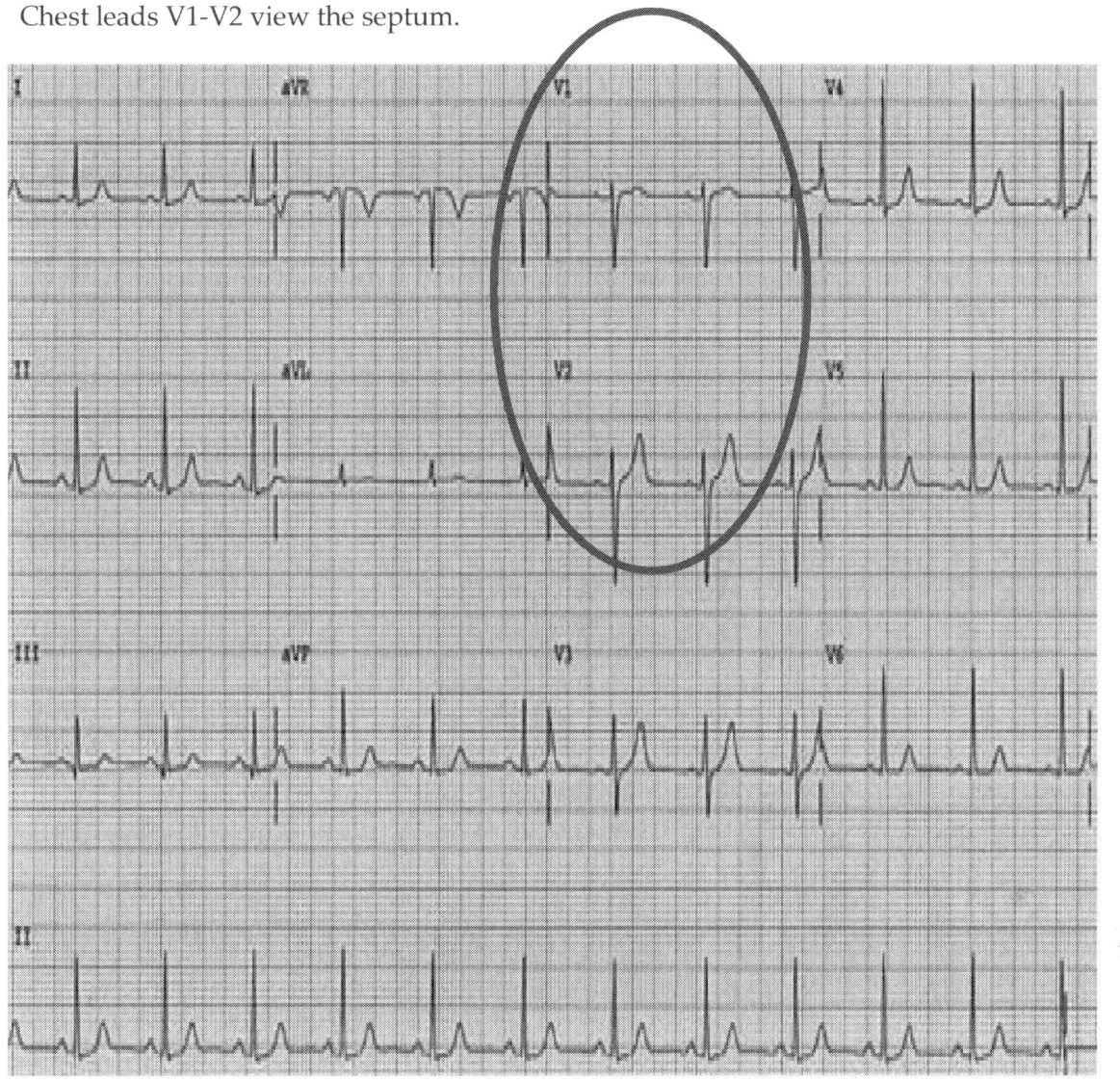

While the most common cause of complete heart block associated with myocardial infarction is occlusion of the right coronary artery, involvement of the septum in left anterior descending coronary artery infarction is particularly ominous as this affects the bundle of His. Injury to the bundle of His may result in abrupt heart block without warning. For this reason, some advocate placement of an external cardiac pacemaker on standby in managing anterior wall myocardial infarction. Chest leads V2-V3-V4 monitor the "anterior wall" of the heart that houses the septal Bundle of His.

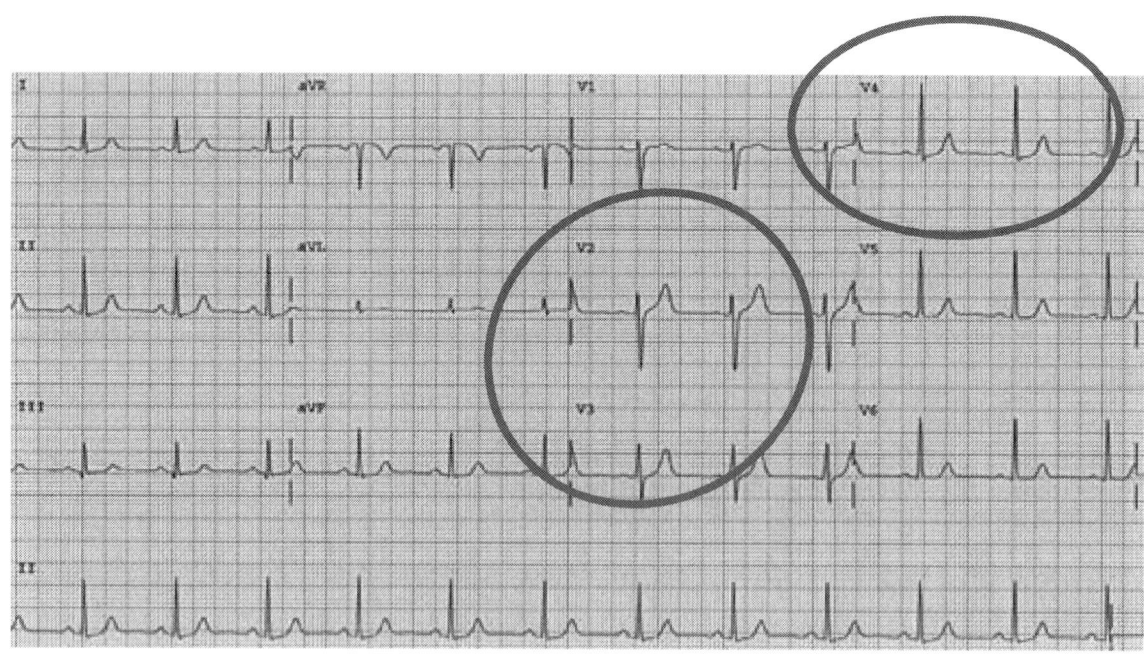

V2-V3-V4 – Anterior Wall with Bundle of His

Chest leads V4-V5-V6 focus on the **lateral wall** of the left ventricle just as do limb leads I- II-aVL. Injury to the left ventricle will demonstrate ischemia and infarction patterns in these leads.

Chest leads focused on the lateral wall of the left ventricle V4-V5-V6

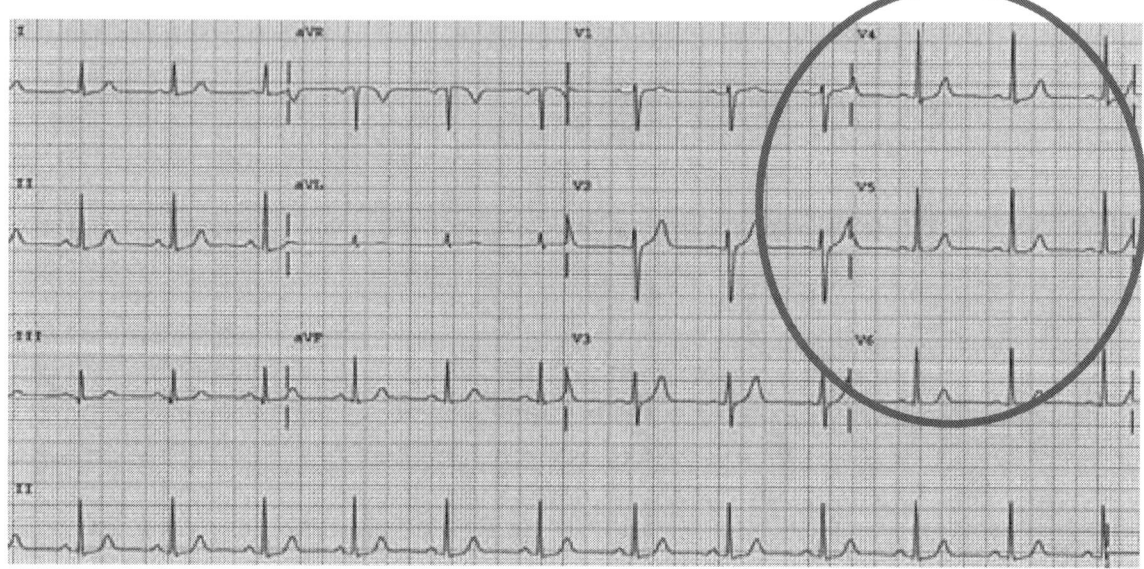

Realize that leads do not possess the same degree of anatomic precision as angiograms. There may be some degree of overlap, particularly with chest leads. While chest lead V2 focuses on the septum, it also sees a portion of the anterior wall of the left ventricle. Likewise, V4 views both the anterior as well as the lateral wall of the left ventricle. V2 and V4 are transitional leads, focusing on both the anterior wall as well as the lateral wall of the left ventricle.

Contiguous Leads in Ischemia and Infarction

Contiguous leads are simply adjacent or adjoining leads. ECG confirmation of either ischemia or infarction must demonstrate characteristic abnormalities in at least *two or more* contiguous leads. The following diagrams illustrate adjacent, i.e., contiguous, limb and chest leads.

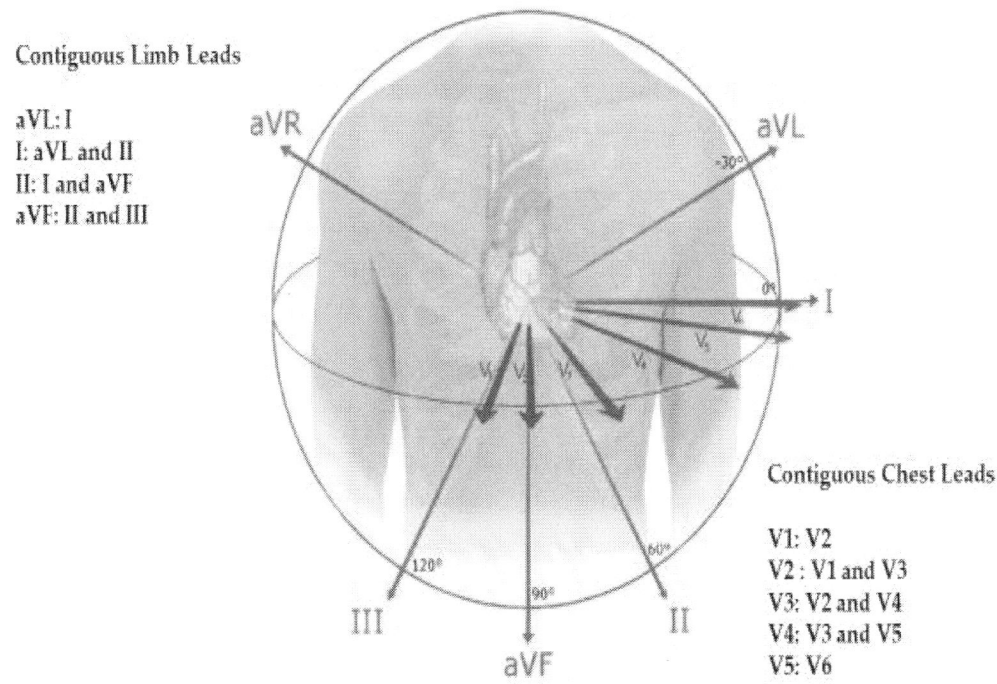

ECG infarction and ischemic patterns should appear in at least two or more adjacent limb and/or chest leads. Appearance in a single lead is suspicious but not diagnostic. Frequently cardiologists refer to such findings as "non-specific changes".

ECG Primary Survey

The Primary Survey aims to identify acute cardiac emergencies rapidly. The actual sequence of the Primary Survey may vary depending on circumstances. For example, signs of cardiogenic shock due to a problematic heart rate demands precedence over searching for ST and T wave abnormalities. Likewise, ventricular rhythms demand intervention prior to other considerations because they are unstable and may quickly degenerate into fatal ventricular fibrillation. In an otherwise stable patient with chest pain, the following sequence suffices in most cases.

ECG Primary Survey – First Element

1. Is heart rate too fast or too slow causing cardiovascular instability?

We have already discussed the importance of patient identifier data. Always be sure that you are looking at the correct ECG!

Calculating Heart Rate

Is heart rate causing cardiovascular instability? In assessing patients with acute chest pain, you need to determine heart rate quickly as well as assess the patient's clinical presentation to answer this question. A cardiac monitor displays heart rate automatically. However, the ability to determine heart rate from a rhythm strip represents a basic ECG skill. You can easily determine heart rate from a rhythm strip with either of the following techniques.

On a rhythm strip, count the number of *large* squares between two consecutive QRS complexes. Then divide 300 by that number. In the example below, there are approximately four large squares between consecutive QRS complexes.

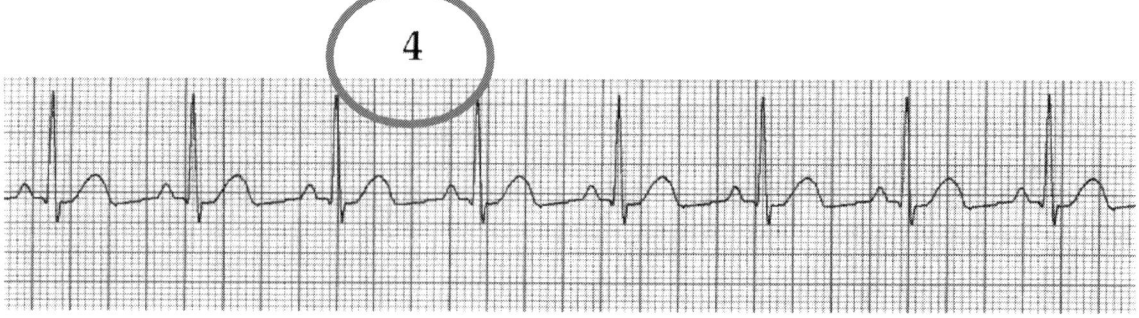

Divide 300 by the number of large spaces: **300/4 = ~ 75.** Why 300? Because each 5 mm large block on the ECG grid represents 0.2 seconds at normal paper speed passing under the machine stylus. If we divide 60 seconds by 0.2, three hundred squares pass beneath the recording stylus in a single minute.

Note that the smallest 1.mm square on the ECG grid represents 0.04 seconds. Five one mm squares comprise a single large 5 mm square. A five mm square represents 0.2 seconds (5 x 0.04).

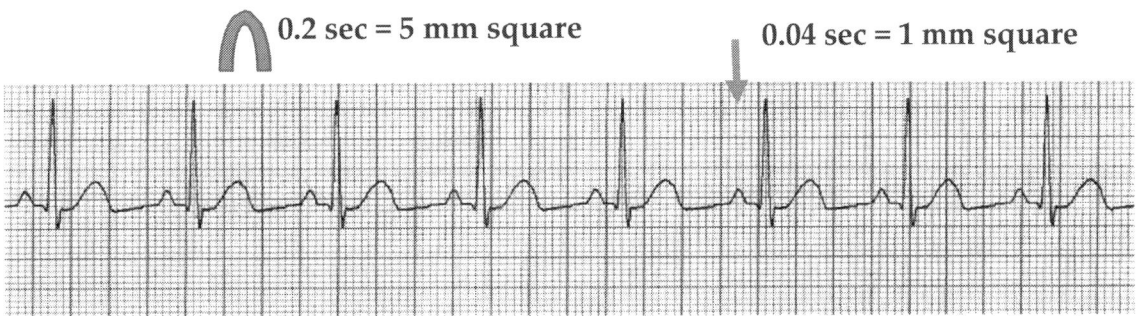

Another rapid method that does not require division assigns the following number sequence from a QRS complex starting point to **each succeeding heavy dividing line** on the ECG grid: **300-150-100-75-60-50-43-37**.

The starting point is any QRS complex that falls on or very near a heavy dividing line. To measure the rate, go to Lead II and locate a QRS complex that is on or closest to a dark line. Start there. Count forward or backwards to the next QRS. whichever line the **next** QRS falls on is the heart rate. Example:

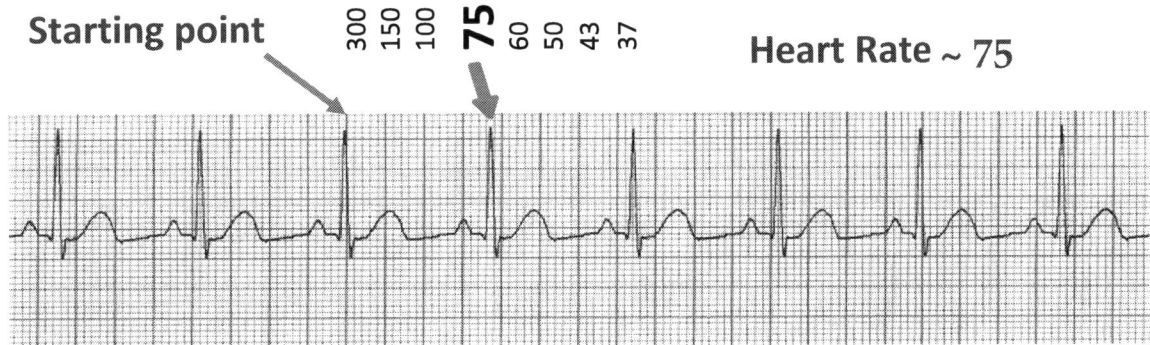

Is heart rate problematic?

Is the heart rate causing cardiovascular instability due to inadequate tissue perfusion?

A runner will exhibit a fast heart rate during exercise. A regular jogger may demonstrate a very slow heart rate at rest. In either case, the heart rate is appropriate in these instances. Neither individual exhibits any sign of physiologic distress or shock. In the examples above, you would expect a fast heart rate when sprinting. Over time in a well-conditioned athlete, the resting heart rate may be low, even in the fifties, due to resetting of the sinoatrial node's intrinsic rate. This results in a larger stroke volume that maintains cardiac output.

Heart rate may be problematic if it is so slow or so fast that heart rate causes "cardiovascular instability" due to inadequate cardiac output. Heart rate may be so fast that the ventricles do not fill adequately or so slow that the ventricular output cannot meet physiologic demand. In the setting of acute cardiac emergencies, such rates may result in inadequate tissue perfusion resulting in cardiogenic shock.

Does the person appear unstable, i.e., is he or she hypotensive – sweaty – diaphoretic – confused? Is the quality of the pulse "thready"? If so, these signs may indicate insufficient cardiac output. Such physical findings require intervention to either slow the rate down or speed the rate up, following current ACLS guidelines.

When confronting a very slow or very fast heart rate that may be problematic, you have to decide whether the heart rate itself is the primary issue. If the rate represents a normal physiologic response to some other factor or condition, *the existing condition requires attention – not the heart rate.* For example, some cardiac medications result in a slower than expected heart rate. Under these circumstances, intervention to speed up the rate is unnecessary. Reducing medication dosage may solve the problem.

EXERCISE– ECG CASE 2

Determine heart rate for each rhythm strip. Complete prior to viewing the video link.

A.

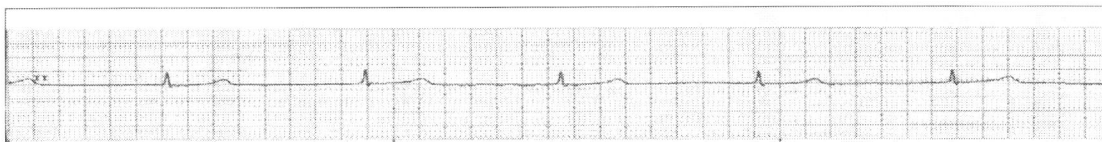

B.

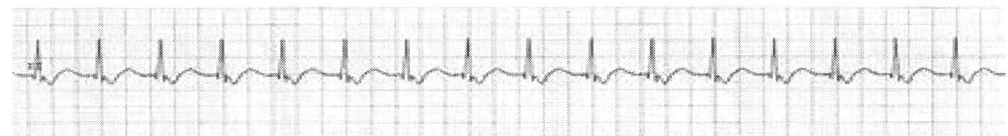

C.

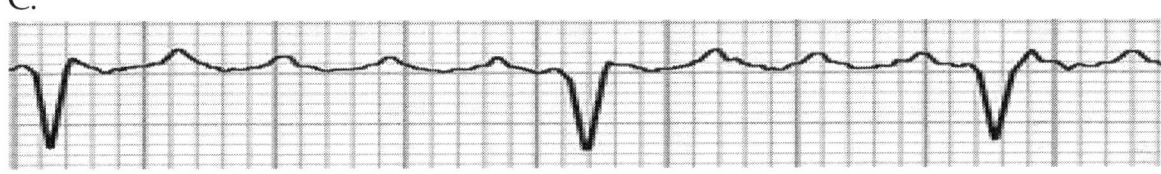

D.

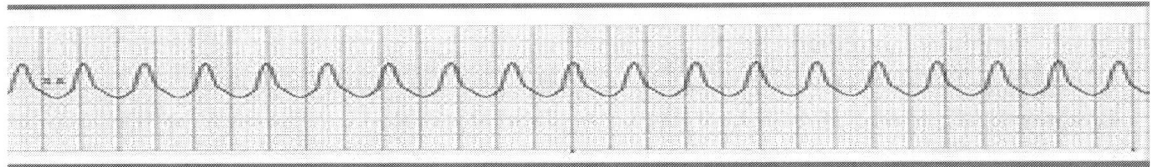

E.

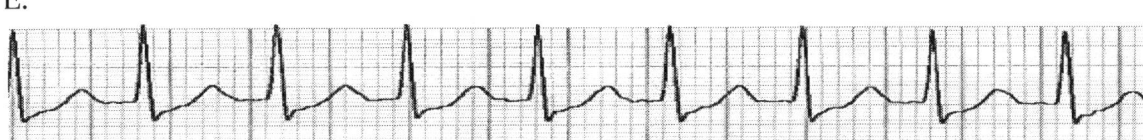

Video Companion link: https://youtu.be/a-fx6Bgylrs

Timestamp 1:11

ECG Primary Survey – Second element

2. Is rhythm supraventricular or ventricular?

More than 1.5 million people suffer myocardial infarction each year in the United States. Cardiac arrhythmias, especially ventricular tachycardia and ventricular fibrillation, may cause sudden death in patients with acute cardiac syndromes.

Ventricular rhythms are inherently unstable. In the setting of acute myocardial infarction, ventricular arrhythmias may result in sudden death if unrecognized and untreated. First responders must decide if the cardiac rhythm is supraventricular or ventricular in origin. To do this, examine the *width* of the QRS complex.

A **narrow** QRS complex is **normal** and indicates a **supraventricular** rhythm, meaning the heart rhythm originates above the ventricles. Such rhythms tend to be stable, although supraventricular rhythms may create problems if sustained over long periods. A **wide** QRS complex is **abnormal** and indicates a **ventricular** rhythm. **Ventricular rhythms are unstable and may deteriorate into sudden ventricular fibrillation or asystole.**

What constitutes a wide QRS complex? A wide QRS complex spans more than **three small (one mm) squares** on the ECG grid:

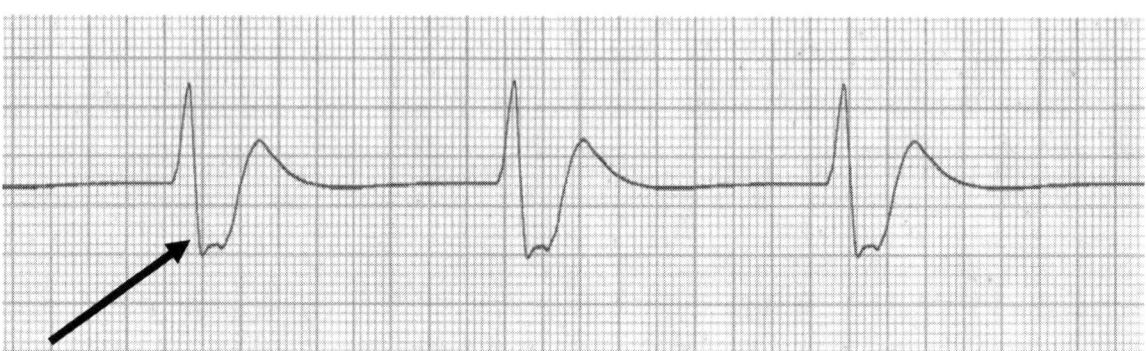

Consider a QRS greater than 3 one mm squares (0.12 seconds) a ventricular beat or ventricular rhythm.

23

Another example of wide QRS

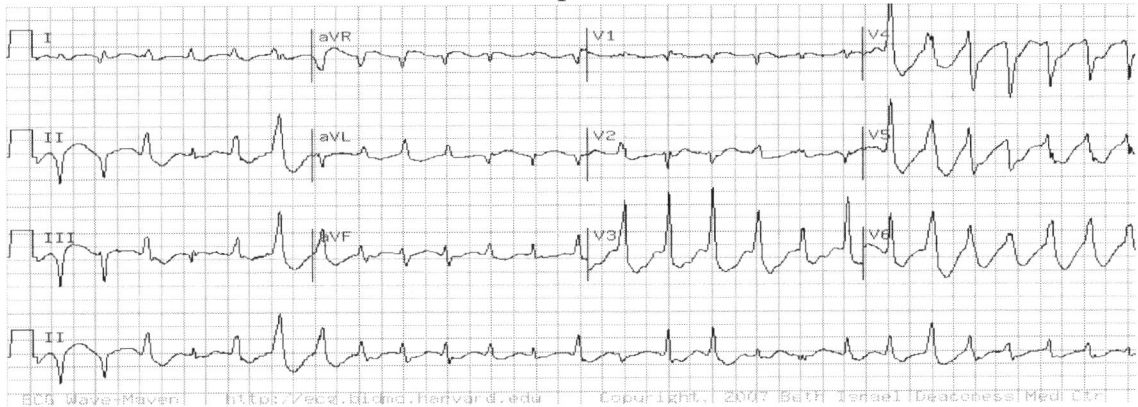

With permission: Nathanson LA, McClennen S, Safran C, Goldberger AL. ECG Wave-Maven: Self-Assessment Program for Students and Clinicians. http://ecg.bidmc.harvard.edu.

AV node blood supply is by a branch of the right coronary artery in 90% of people. Complete AV block, characterized by non-propagated atrial beats resulting in independent, unrelated atrial and ventricular rhythms is most commonly seen in right coronary artery occlusion and inferior MI. Patients with third degree AV block typically experience severe bradycardia, hypotension, and at times, hemodynamic instability due to inadequate tissue perfusion.

A particularly ominous ventricular arrhythmia in the setting of left anterior descending myocardial infarction is third degree heart block that may appear abruptly without warning. In such situations, first responders must be prepared to initiate external cardiac pacing on standby.

Other conditions may cause widening of the QRS complex, such as bundle branch blocks, creating a "pseudo-ventricular" appearing rhythm. In these cases, the cardiac electrical impulse does not follow its usual conduction path through the bundle of His but rather a circuitous route that results in a widened QRS. Unless you have received advanced ECG training in bundle branch block recognition, you should assume that a wide QRS represents a ventricular arrhythmia in the setting of acute chest pain. In such situations, be prepared to follow your training in ACLS for management of ventricular arrhythmias.

Because fatal cardiac arrhythmias occur commonly in ischemia and infarction, patients require continuous cardiac monitoring beginning on-scene, during transport, and throughout their hospital stay. Although 12 lead ECG includes a rhythm strip, the 12 lead ECG records a static picture of cardiac activity – a single moment in time. Only continuous cardiac monitoring can detect potentially lethal cardiac arrhythmias as they develop.

ECG Primary Survey – Third element

3. Are ST segments consistent with STEMI / NSTEMI?

Scan the ECG for abnormal ST segments, the key to diagnose myocardial ischemia or infarction. Although the ST segment appears as an inconspicuous part of the QRS complex, its migration from the baseline, known as the "isoelectric" line, indicates infarction if elevated or ischemia if depressed.

A normal ST segment should always fall on the isoelectric line.

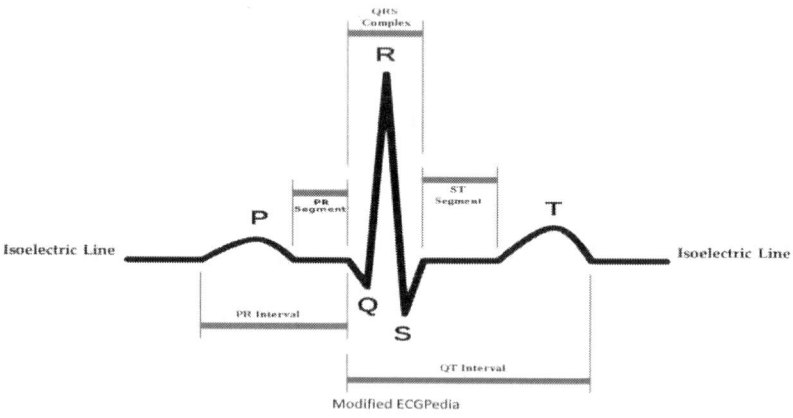

ST Segment in Myocardial Infarction

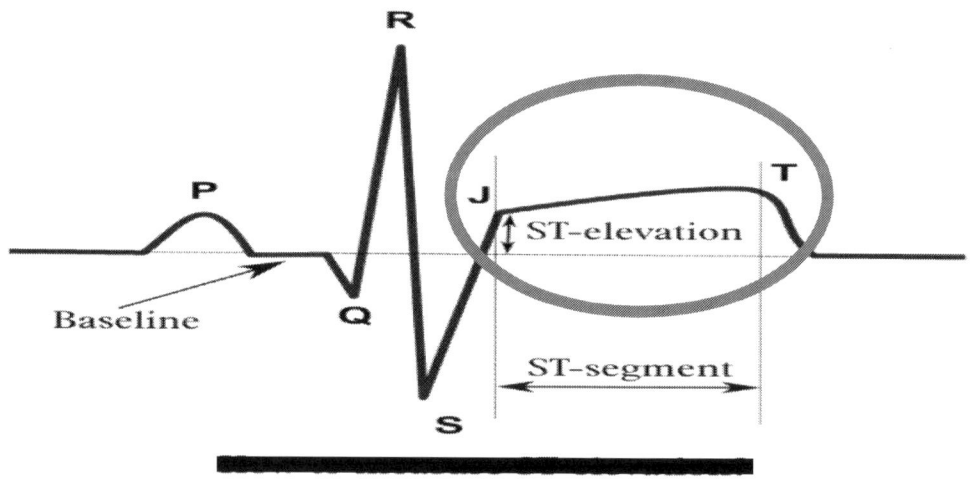

In myocardial infarction, the ST segment rises **ABOVE** the baseline of the tracing. You should scan ST segments in **EVERY** lead, both limb and chest. The height of ST segment will vary depending on the extent of the infarction. The greater the elevation, the more extensive the infarct.

Early Benign Repolarization – J Point Elevation

The J point marks the end of the S wave and the beginning of the ST segment. Widespread ST elevation secondary to a high J point takeoff may mimic STEMI. However, careful examination of the shape of the ST segment in such instances reveals a "concave" appearance, unlike the convex shape associated with STEMI, sometimes referred to as "tombstoning". With STEMI, the convex shape assumes a "frowny" face appearance, whereas with high J point elevation, the convex ST segment assumes a "smiley" face.

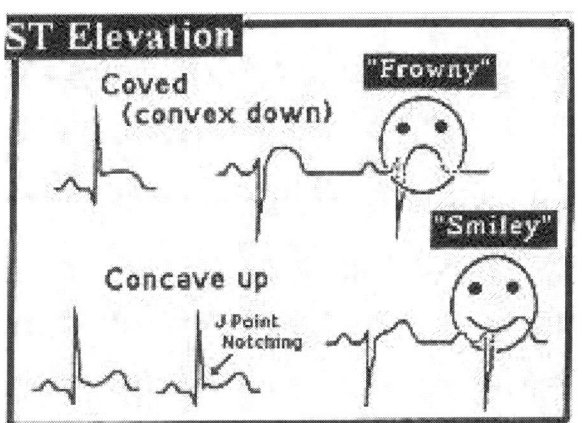 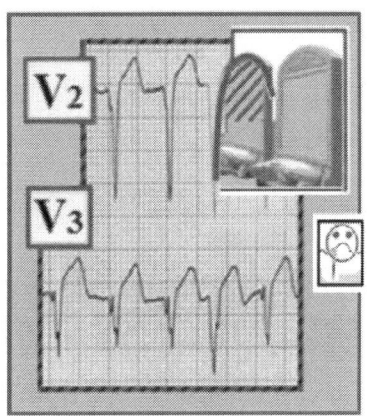

Reproduced with permission from Ken Grauer, MD from ECG-2014-ePub (KG/EKG Press Dr. Grauer's ECG Interpretation Blog)

J point elevation represents benign early repolarization (BER) and is commonly seen in young, healthy patients less than 50 years of age. It produces widespread ST segment elevation, most prominently in precordial leads. As many as 10-15% of patients presenting with chest pain may have BER on their ECG, making it a diagnostic challenge to distinguish between STEMI and benign early repolarization.

ST Segment in Myocardial Ischemia

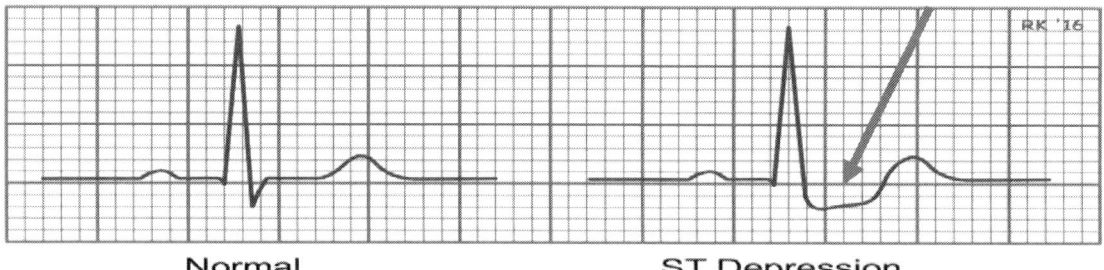

Reproduced with permission Richard E. Klabunde, PhD

In myocardial ischemia, ST segments fall **BELOW** the baseline of the tracing (green arrow). You should scan ST segments in **EVERY** lead, both limb and chest.

ECG Primary Survey – Fourth Element

4. Are T waves consistent with STEMI / NSTEMI?

T waves represent ventricular repolarization. Normal T waves appear as positive or upright deflections following the ST segment in all leads except aVR, where the entire QRS-T wave complex is inverted. Any limb or chest lead that sees the depolarization approaching will have upright QRS-T wave complexes. Conversely, any lead that sees the depolarization moving away will have inverted QRS-T wave complexes, viz., aVR. Thus, all limb leads except aVR will exhibit upright QRS-T wave complexes. Chest leads V2 through V6 will have upright T wave complexes. The R wave in the QRS complex in chest leads will become increasingly taller from V1 through V6.

In STEMI and NSTEMI, T waves are **inverted**. However, sometimes, elevated ST segments may mask T wave inversion.

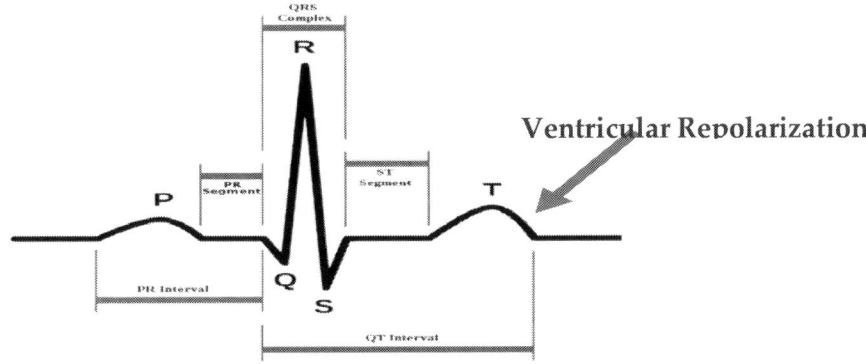

T wave height or amplitude is normally less than 5 mm in limb leads and less than 15 mm in chest leads. Many conditions may affect the appearance of T waves. Flat T waves appear in hypokalemia. In hyperkalemia, T waves are tall and peaked. With chest pain in an adult, inverted T waves suggest STEMI if associated with elevated ST segment or NSTEMI if associated with ST segment depression.

How can you distinguish between T wave inversions seen in ischemia from T wave inversions seen in NSTMI, since T wave inversion is present in both conditions? Serum troponin will be elevated in NSTEMI but not in ischemia. Because serum troponin is not available on scene, assume NSTEMI as the cause of T wave inversion rather than ischemia.

Scan **EVERY** lead for T wave inversion with the exception of aVR and V1 where T wave inversion is normal. Symmetric T wave inversion greater than 3 mm (3 small squares on the ECG grid) is abnormal. When present in *two or more adjoining leads*, T wave inversions with abnormal ST segments in the setting of acute chest pain signifies STEMI / NSTEMI until proven otherwise by measurement of serum troponin.

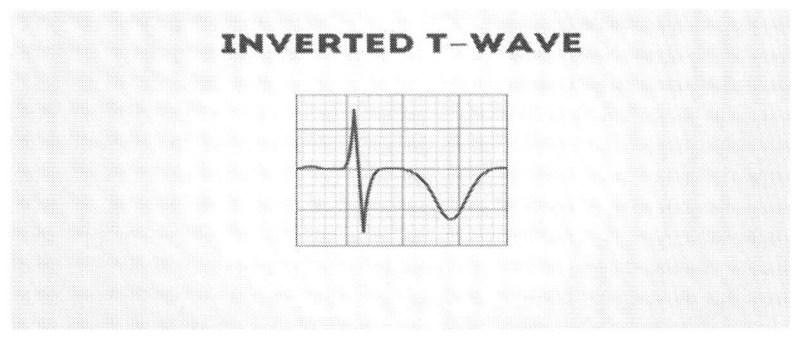

T Wave Inversion. With Permission Dr. Potter.GeekyMedics

Acute Coronary Syndromes – STEMI, NSTEMI and Unstable Angina

ECG leads can identify not only the presence of ischemia and myocardial infarction but also where in the heart injury is occurring. Localization of myocardial injury identifies what coronary artery is involved. This is clinically significant because each coronary artery may present specific and unique challenges in patient management.

Coronary Arteries

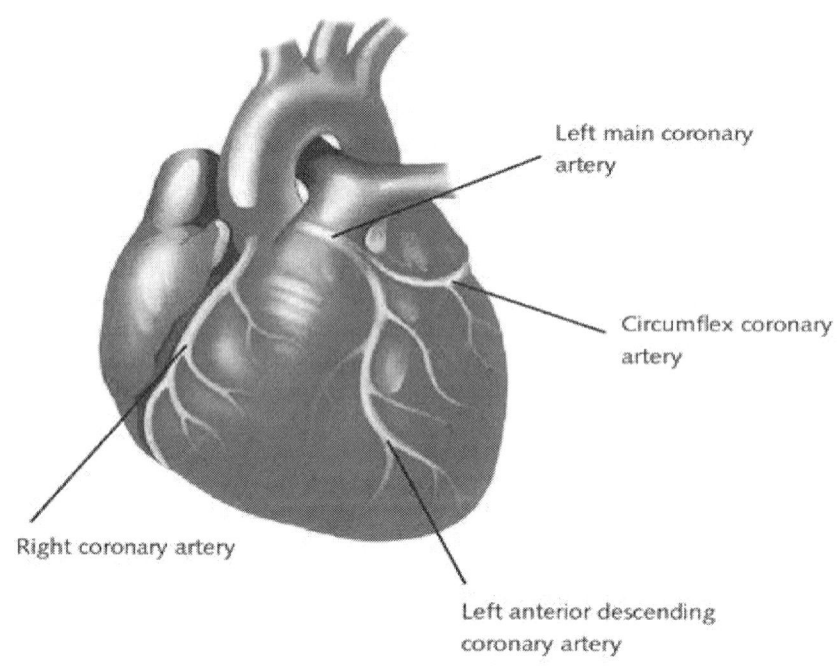

Right coronary artery – Supplies the right ventricle, aka, inferior wall. In 80-85% of cases, the right coronary artery also supplies the posterior descending coronary artery, referred to as right coronary artery dominance.

Left main coronary artery – two branches:

> **Left anterior descending coronary artery** – branch of the left main coronary artery; supplies the anterior wall of the left ventricle and 2/3 of the septum

> **Circumflex artery** – branch of the left main coronary artery; supplies the lateral wall of the left ventricle and, in 10% of cases, supplies the posterior descending coronary artery, referred to as left coronary artery dominance. In the remaining 20% of cases, both right and left coronary arteries anastomose to supply the posterior descending coronary artery, referred to as co-dominance.

STEMI – ST Segment Elevation Myocardial Infarction

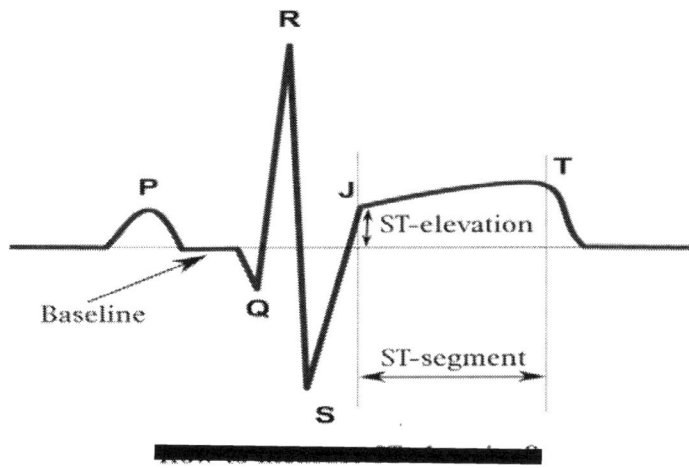

Chest pain with elevated ST segments in two anatomically contiguous (adjacent) leads on ECG and elevated serum troponin confirms the diagnosis of myocardial infarction. However, a normal appearing ECG and normal serum troponin *do not exclude* this diagnosis when patient history and symptoms suggest myocardial injury. In very early stages of infarction, the initial ECG and serum troponin *may be normal*. In such instances, serial ECGs and troponin levels will be necessary to confirm the diagnosis.

Be aware, certain patient populations present with atypical symptoms!

- Atypical presentation may present with non-chest pain symptoms, such as weakness, nausea, sweating, cough, dyspnea, pain in the back, jaw, or head.

- Females, elderly individuals, and those with diabetes often present with atypical symptoms.
- Keep your index of suspicion for ischemia and/or myocardial infarction high when evaluating such patients and err on the side of caution when deciding whether to perform a 12-lead ECG.

STEMI Localization

The Primary Survey identifies **four** STEMI locations to identify the involved coronary arteries:

1. **Inferior wall STEMI** - Right ventricle ⇨ right coronary artery
2. **Anterior Wall STEMI** – Anterior wall of the left ventricle ⇨ left anterior descending coronary artery
3. **Lateral Wall STEMI** - Lateral wall of the left ventricle ⇨ circumflex coronary artery
4. **Posterior Wall STEMI** – Posterior myocardial wall ⇨ posterior descending branch from the right coronary artery in 80% of individuals or branch from the circumflex coronary artery in the remaining 20%.

ECG - Inferior Wall STEMI - Right Coronary Artery

STEMI in limb leads II-aVF-III indicates myocardial infarction involving the diaphragmatic surface of the left ventricle and distal septum, and perhaps a small portion of the right ventricle due to obstruction of blood flow through the **right coronary artery**. The term "inferior wall" refers to the anatomic relationship of the right ventricle to the left ventricle within the chest cavity. The right ventricle lies somewhat beneath or "inferior" to the left ventricular chamber as shown with arrows.

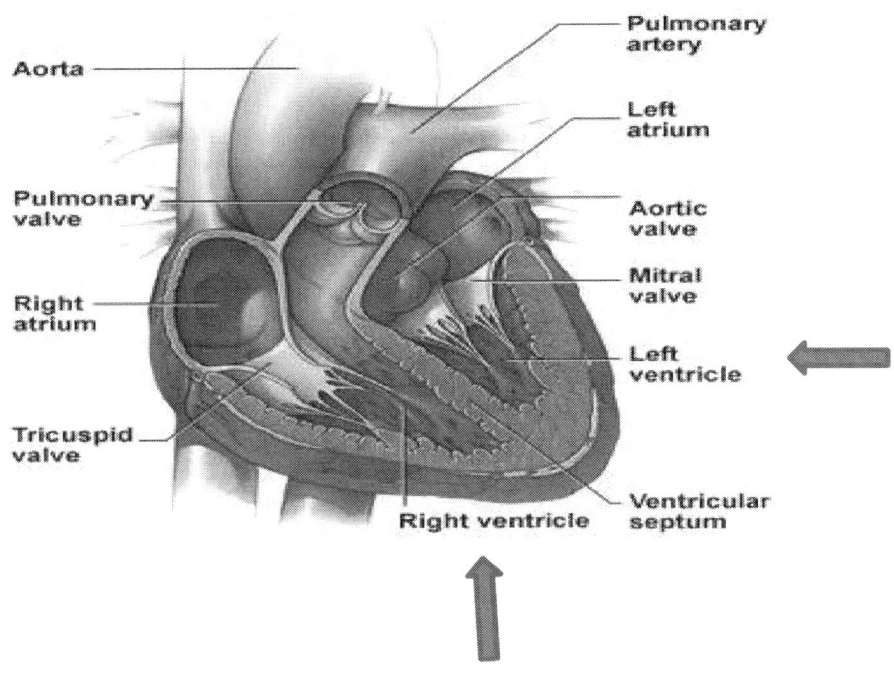

Limb Leads Focused on the Right Ventricle
II –III - aVF

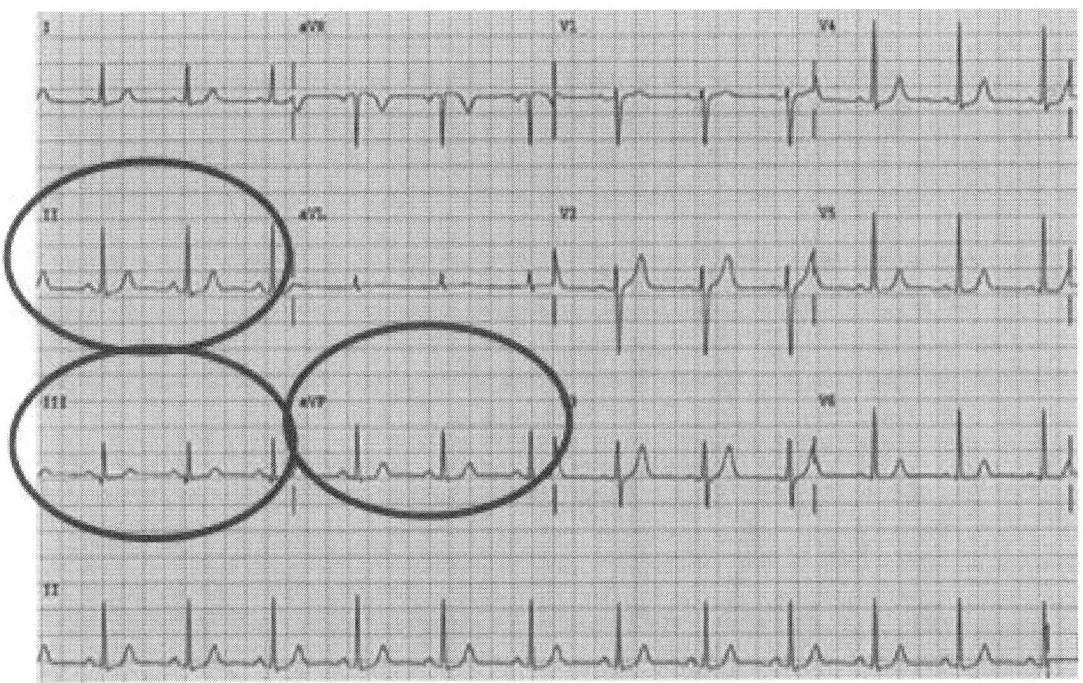

STEMI in limb leads II – III – aVF – Right Ventricle

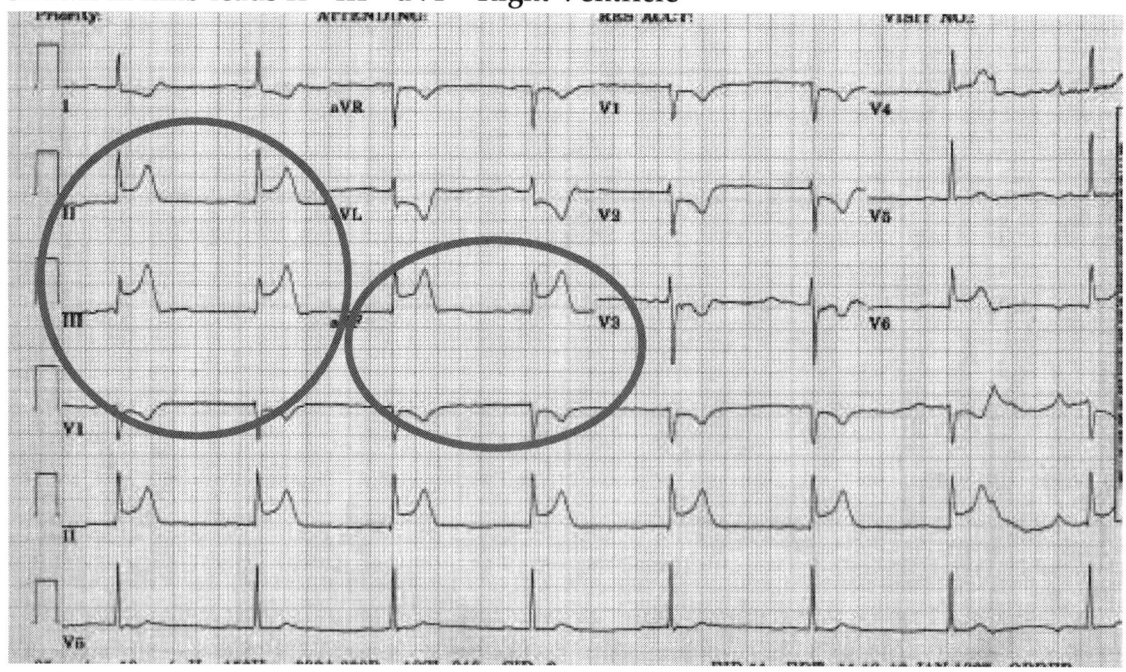

In patients experiencing an inferior wall STEMI, use of phosphodiesterase inhibitors such as tadalafil (Cialis®), sildenafil (Viagra®), vardenafil (Lavitra®), within the previous 24-48 hours, poses a relative contraindication to nitroglycerin administration for chest pain relief. Nitroglycerin causes peripheral blood vessels to dilate. In turn, this reduces the amount of blood flowing into the right ventricle referred to as "preload". Reduction in right ventricular blood flow reduces blood flow into the left ventricle, leading to a reduction in left ventricle filling. Stroke volume becomes less thereby reducing coronary artery blood flow.

ECG – Anterior Wall STEMI - Left Anterior Descending Coronary Artery

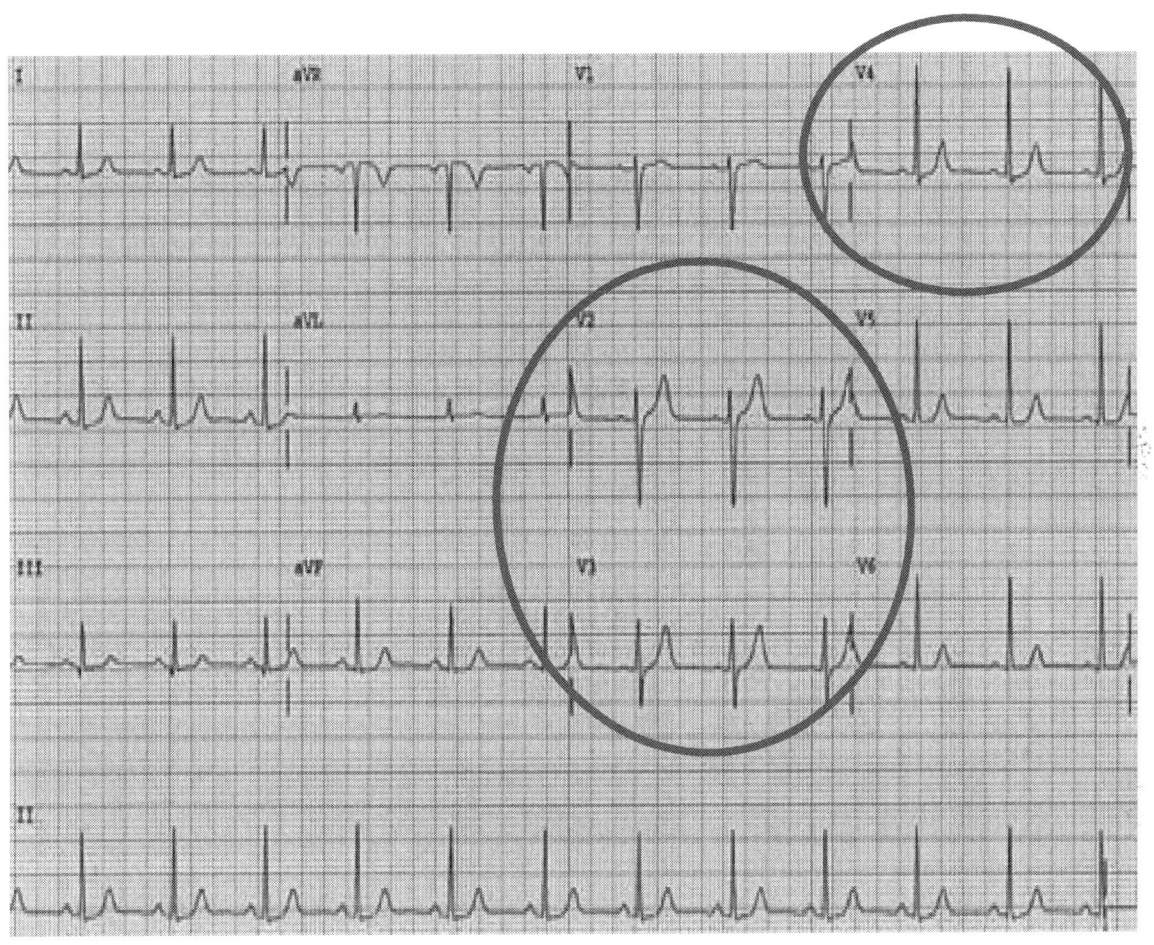

Chest leads focused on the anterior wall of the left ventricle V2-V3-V4

STEMI in Chest Leads V2-V3-V4

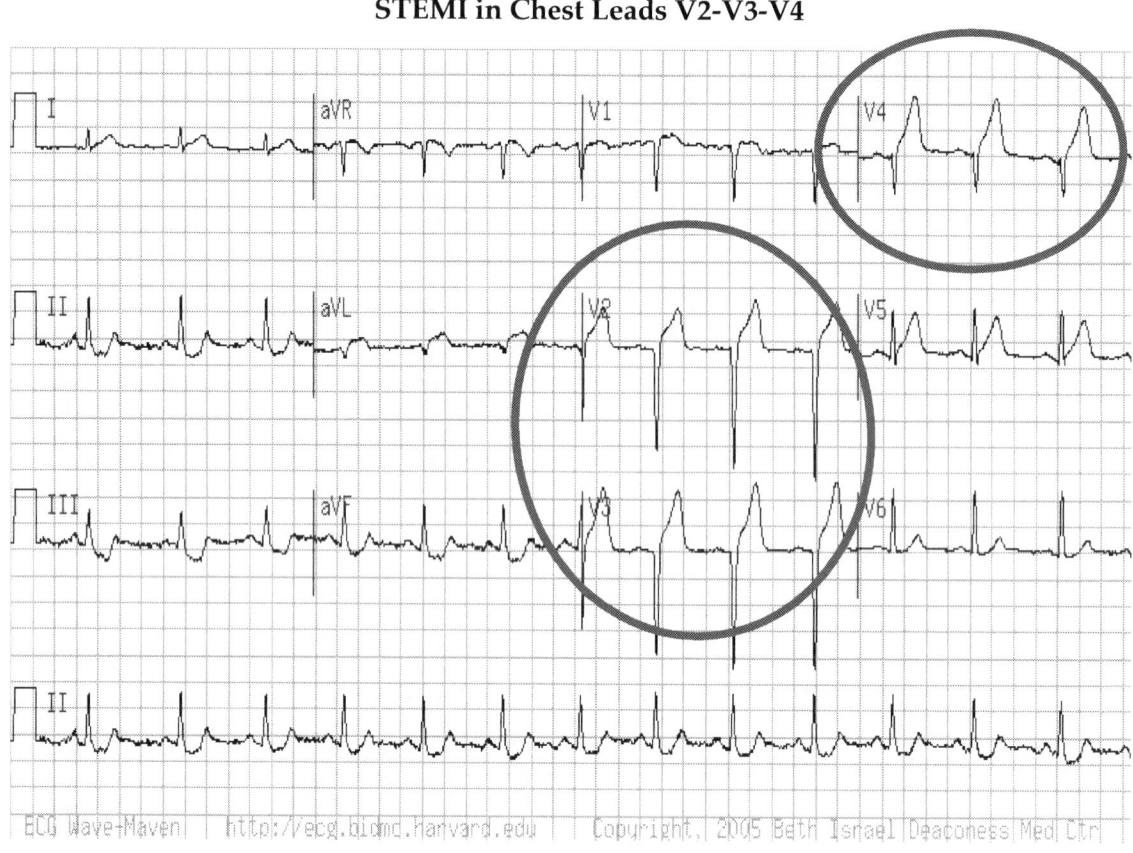

With Permission: Nathanson LA, McClennen S, Safran C, Goldberger AL. ECG Wave-Maven: Self-Assessment Program for Students and Clinicians. http://ecg.bidmc.harvard.edu.

The **left anterior descending coronary artery (LAD)** supplies as much as 45-55% blood to the anterior wall of the left ventricle and 2/3 of the septum's blood supply. Commonly referred to as the "widow maker", stenosis of the LAD may cause sudden 3rd degree heart block due to affected Bundle of His as well as sudden death secondary to ventricular fibrillation. Immediate percutaneous coronary intervention (PCI) to re-establish coronary artery blood flow remains the treatment of choice to survive this devastating event. With sudden onset of 3rd degree heart block, transcutaneous pacing may serve as a bridge to emergent transvenous pacing.

ECG – Lateral Wall STEMI - Circumflex Coronary Artery

The circumflex coronary artery, branching from the left main coronary artery, supplies the lateral wall of the left ventricle. Remember that both limb leads I-II-aVL and chest leads V4-V5-V6 focus on the left ventricle.

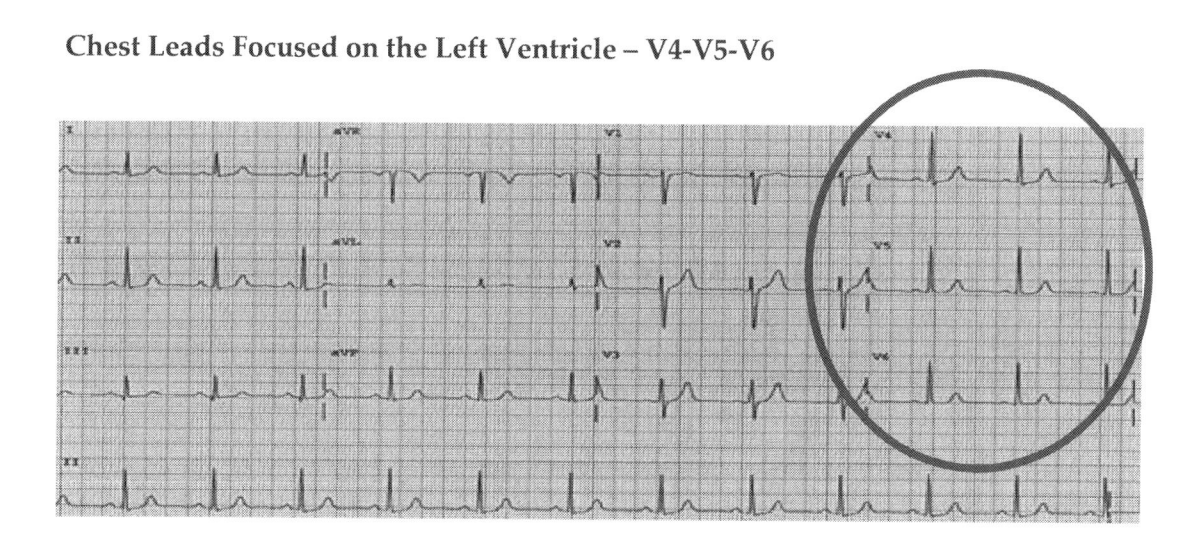

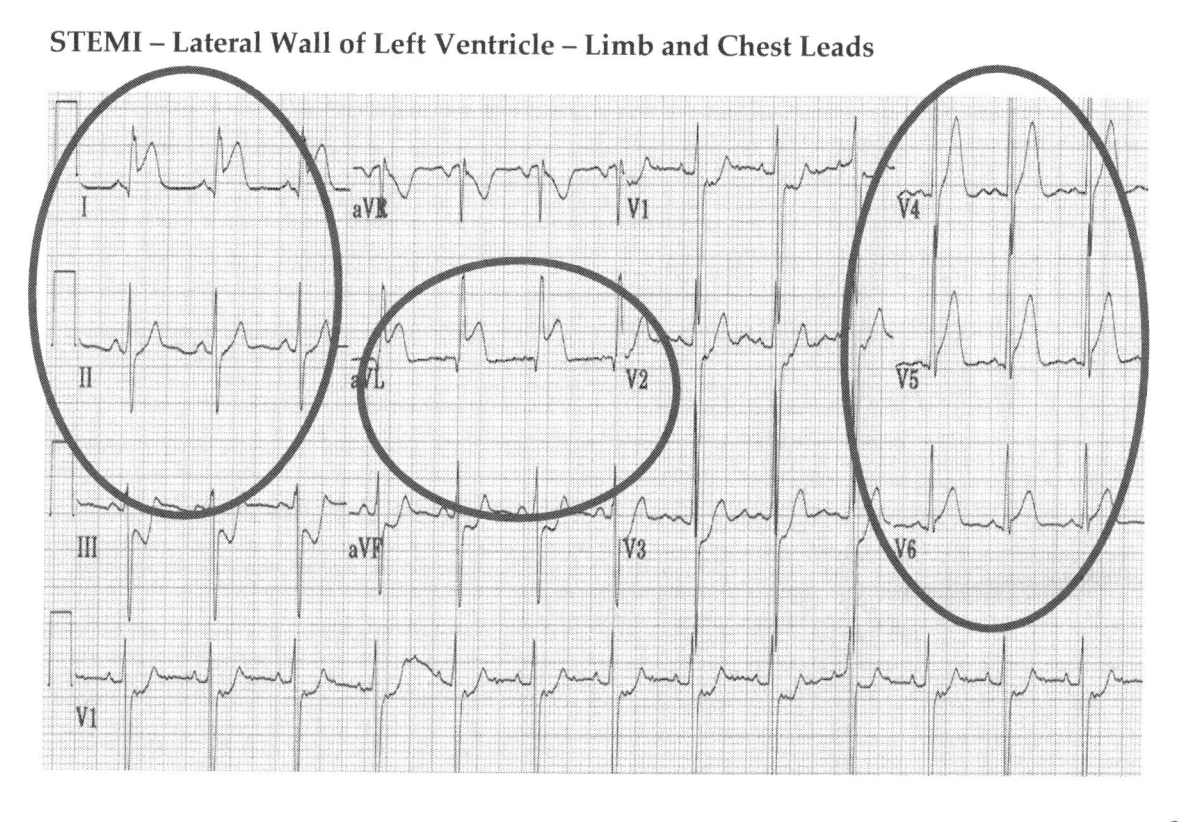

Chest Leads Focused on the Left Ventricle – V4-V5-V6

STEMI – Lateral Wall of Left Ventricle – Limb and Chest Leads

An occlusion occurring in the left main coronary artery, *prior to its bifurcation*, will affect both left anterior descending and circumflex branches. ST segment elevation will occur across chest leads V2 through V6, indicating a significant and extensive myocardial injury, referred to as an "antero-lateral" myocardial infarction.

ST Segment elevation in limb leads I-II-aVL and chest leads V2-V3-V4-V5-V6 Antero-lateral STEMI

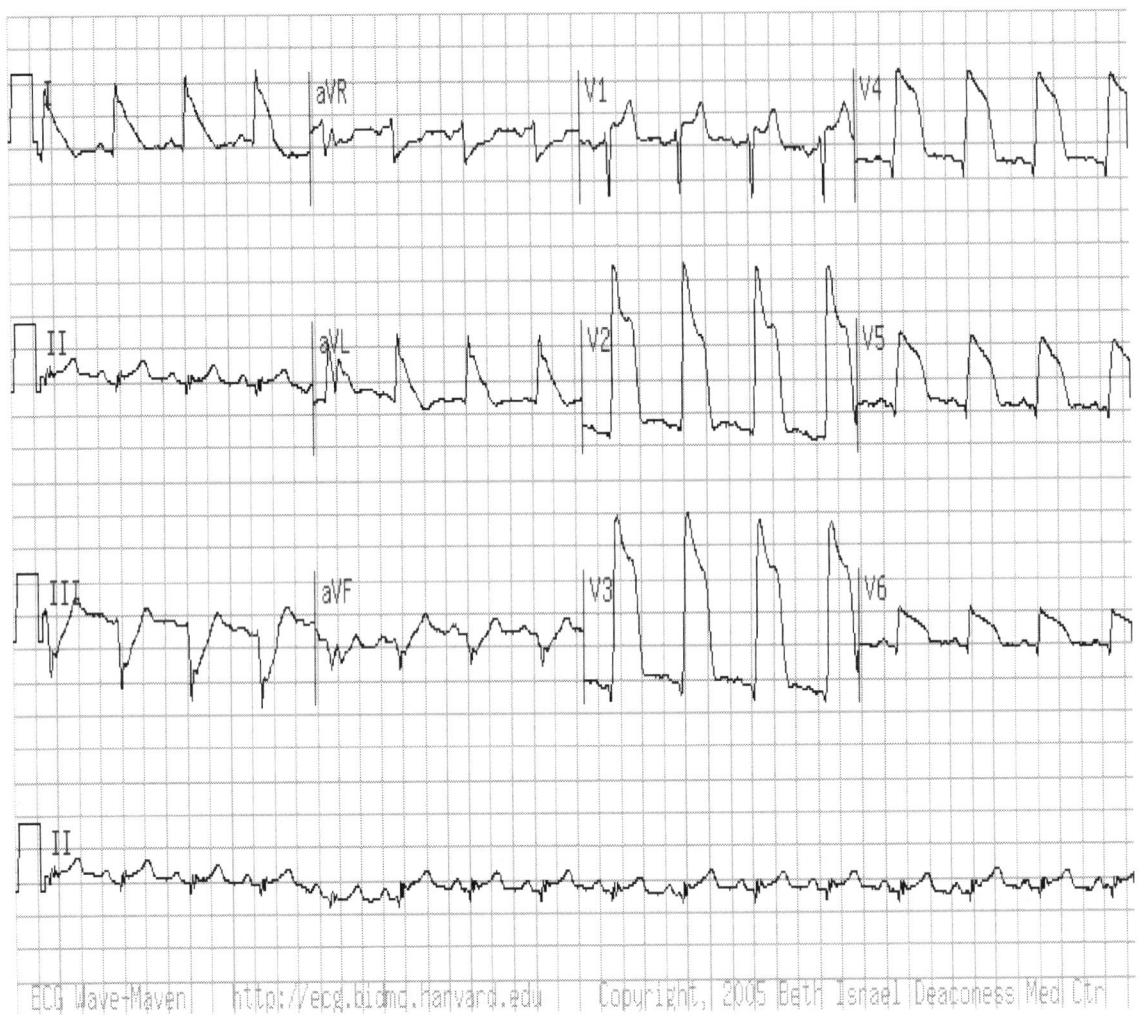

With Permission: Nathanson LA, McClennen S, Safran C, Goldberger AL. ECG Wave-Maven: Self-Assessment Program for Students and Clinicians.
http://ecg.bidmc.harvard.edu.

Posterior Wall STEMI – ECG Blind Spot

Posterior wall STEMI represents the "blind spot" on the 12 lead ECG. Because the standard 12 lead ECG does not position any electrodes on the left side of the chest posteriorly, a STEMI involving the posterior descending coronary artery, also known as the posterior interventricular artery, will not appear in any lead as ST segment elevation and T wave inversion, the classic STEMI configuration. Instead, a posterior STEMI appears as ST segment DEPRESSION followed by an UPRIGHT T wave in chest leads V1-V2-V3 and dominant R wave in V2-V3 (R/S ratio > 1). Such changes reflect an inverted appearance of the QRS-T wave complex normally seen with an acute infarction.

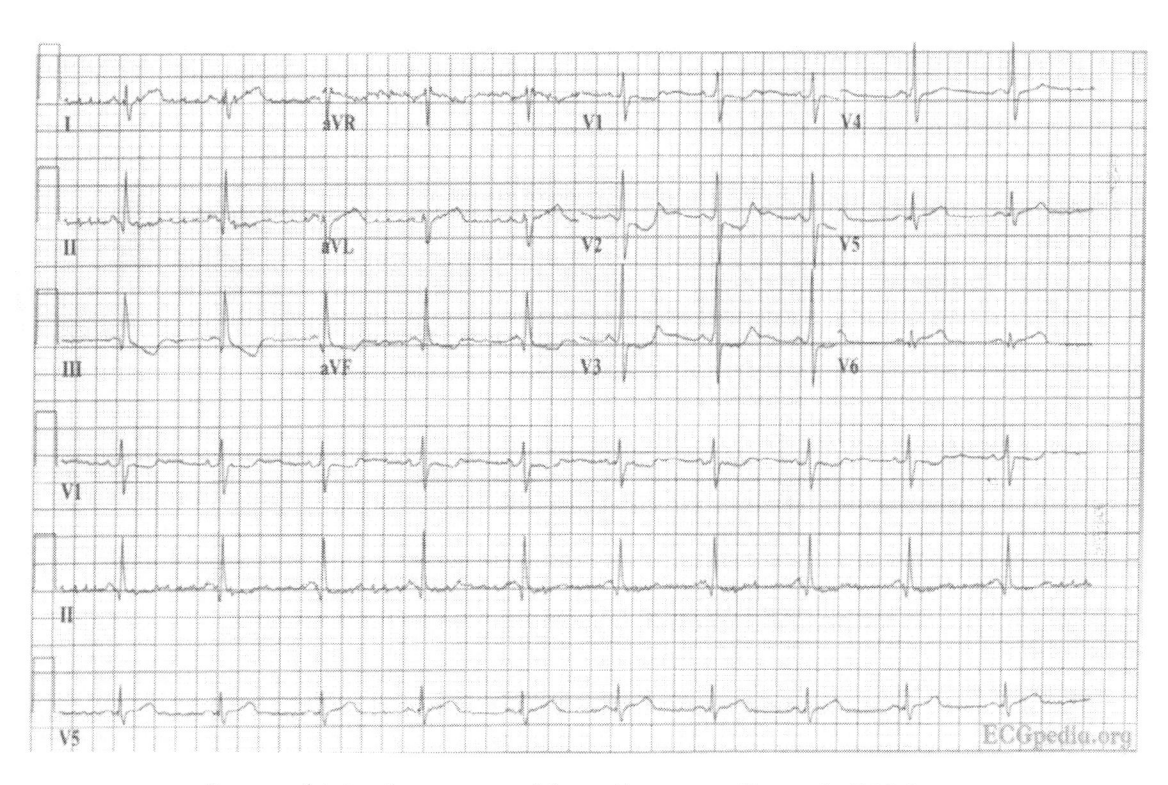

Image obtained courtesy of, http://en.ecgpedia.org/wiki/Main

This inverted QRS-T wave complex represents a "reciprocal change" as explained by the following. The normal direction the electrical wave of depolarization travels is from right to left diagonally, i.e., SA node – AV node – His bundle - Purkinje fibers – ventricles. Any electrode in the path of the oncoming wave will show upright QRS complexes. Likewise, any electrode that sees the wave moving away will record downward deflections. Lead aVR sees the depolarization wave moving away and, therefore, records an inverted QRS-T wave pattern. All the other limb leads see the wave approaching and record upright QRS-T wave patterns on the ECG.

Electrical Wave of Depolarization from Right to Left Diagonally

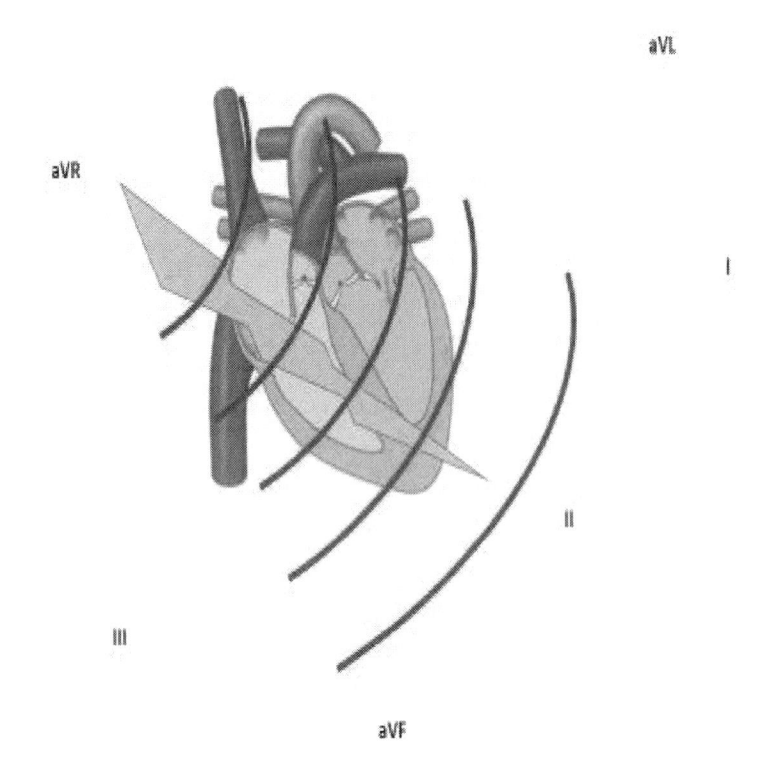

Opposing Limb Leads and Reciprocal Changes

Lead aVR is directly opposite lead II. Because aVR sees the depolarization moving away, the QRS-T wave is inverted. Because the remaining limb leads see the depolarization approaching, the QRS-T wave patterns are upright, with the tallest QRS complex appearing in lead II. This lead reflects the full force of the depolarization wave and therefore shows the most positive, i.e., upright, QRS among limb leads. These opposing patterns represent "reciprocal changes".

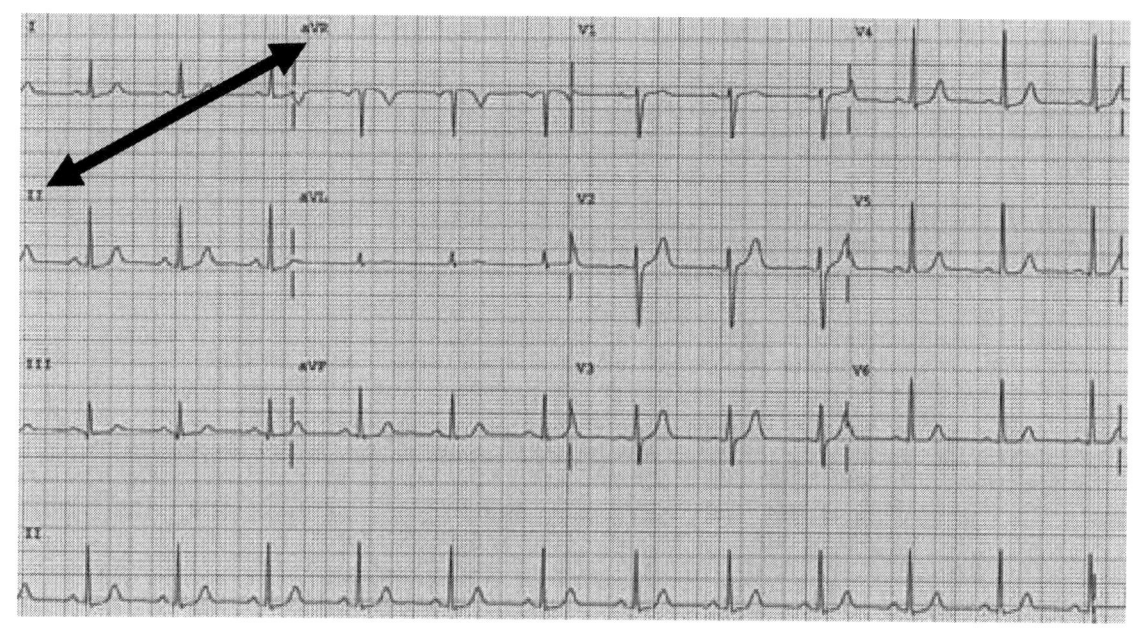

Reciprocal leads II and aVR

Recall that chest leads view the heart in a cross-sectional plane. In a posterior wall STEMI, anterior chest leads V1-V2-V3 become reciprocal leads and therefore will demonstrate ST segment depression and upright T waves instead of ST elevation and T wave inversion as seen in STEMI. If we position ECG electrodes posteriorly as shown below, the ECG will then demonstrate the classic ST segment elevation-T wave inversion characteristic of infarction.

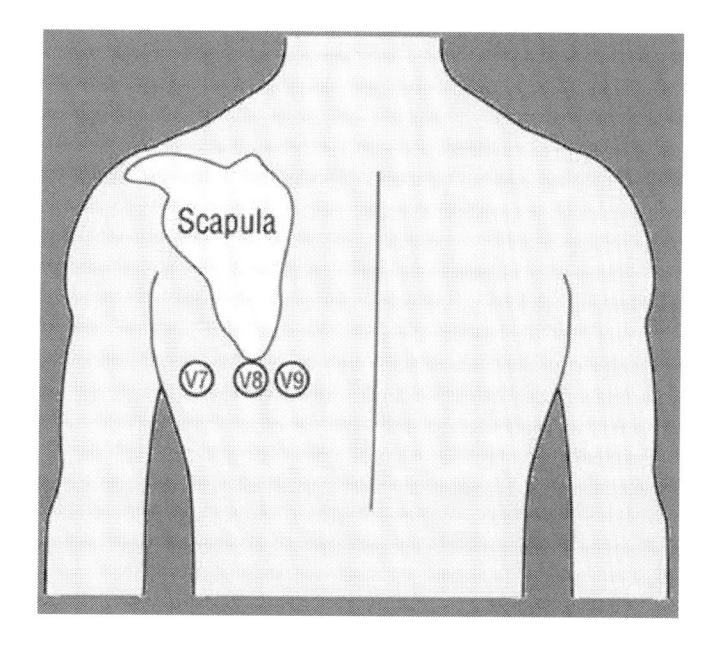

https://sites.google.com/site/electrocardiologyinstruction/

In patients presenting with ischemic symptoms, ST segment depression in V1-V2-V3 with upright T waves should immediately raise concerns for a posterior STEMI and not regarded as merely ischemia. However, unless you remember to look for such changes, you will easily miss this diagnosis. Thus, the so-called "ECG blind spot"!

Localization of NSTEMI

The localization of NSTEMI mirrors that in STEMI, i.e., a NSTEMI in the right coronary artery demonstrates ECG ischemic patterns in limb leads II, III, and aVF in patients who are right coronary artery dominant (80-85%). NSTEMI ECG changes involving the LAD will appear primarily in chest leads V2-V4, while NSTEMI in the left circumflex coronary artery appears in limb leads I, II, aVL and chest leads V5-V6.

In this ECG, notice the T wave inversions in limb leads I, II, aVF and chest leads as well as ST segment depression in chest leads V3, V4, V5. In addition, there is T wave inversion in V6.

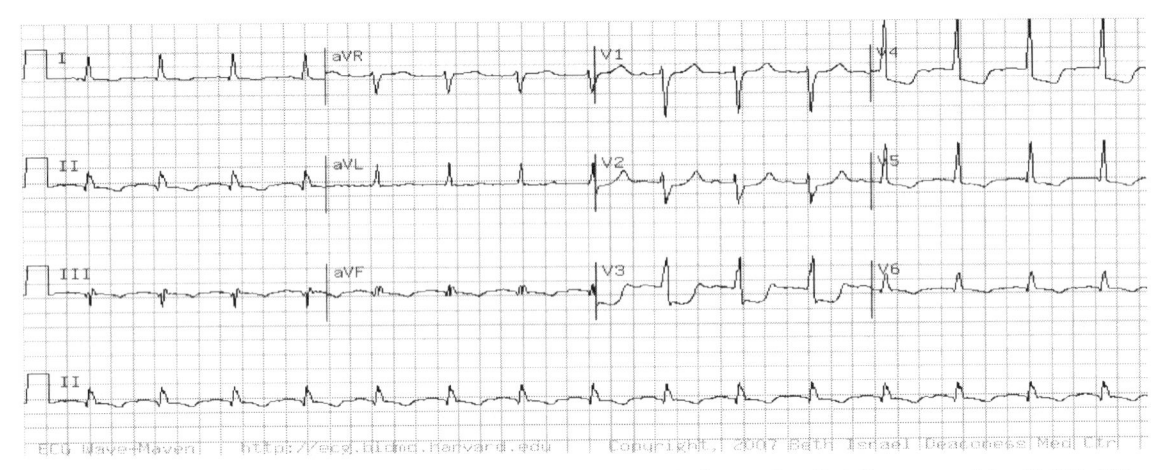

With Permission: Nathanson LA, McClennen S, Safran C, Goldberger AL. ECG Wave-Maven: Self-Assessment Program for Students and Clinicians.
http://ecg.bidmc.harvard.edu.

T wave inversions in limb leads II, III, aVF signify right coronary artery involvement, while the ST segment depressions in chest leads V2-V5 implicates the left anterior descending coronary artery. Since both arteries appear involved, interference with coronary artery blood flow appears extensive. These changes may be either a NSTEMI or unstable angina, depending on whether or not serum troponin is elevated. In the field, such changes mandate NSTEMI alert pending completion of troponin levels at the receiving medical care facility.

SUMMARY STEMI AND NSTEMI LOCALIZATION

Limb Leads	
aVL	
I	**Lateral Wall**
II	
II	
aVF	**Inferior Wall**
III	

Chest Leads	
V1	
	Septum / Posterior
	Wall V2
V3	
	Anterior Wall
V4	
V5	
	Lateral Wall V6

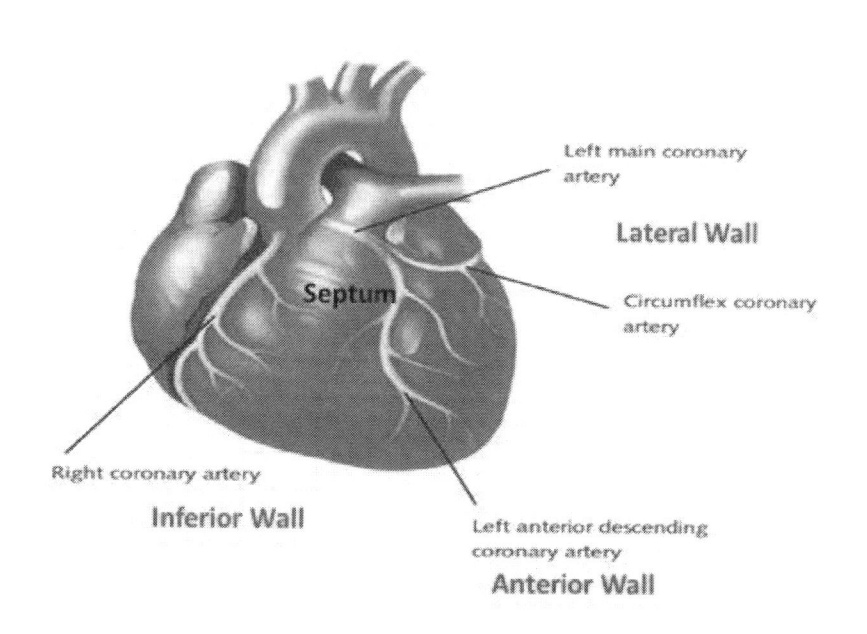

Left main coronary artery

Lateral Wall

Septum

Circumflex coronary artery

Right coronary artery

Inferior Wall

Left anterior descending coronary artery

Anterior Wall

Ischemia versus NSTEMI: ST Segment and T waves

Non-ST elevation myocardial infarction (NSTEMI) indicates a partial occlusion of a coronary vessel as opposed to total occlusion in STEMI. As with STEMI, this partial occlusion will cause elevation of serum troponin, indicative of cardiac injury.

Ischemia may present with similar ECG findings of ST segment depression and T wave inversion. Because first responders will not know if serum troponin is elevated, assume ST SEGMENT DEPRESSION below the isoelectric baseline and T WAVE INVERSIONS as indicative of NSTEMI. In addition, findings suggestive of ischemia on ECG will not show reciprocal changes as seen with STEMI.

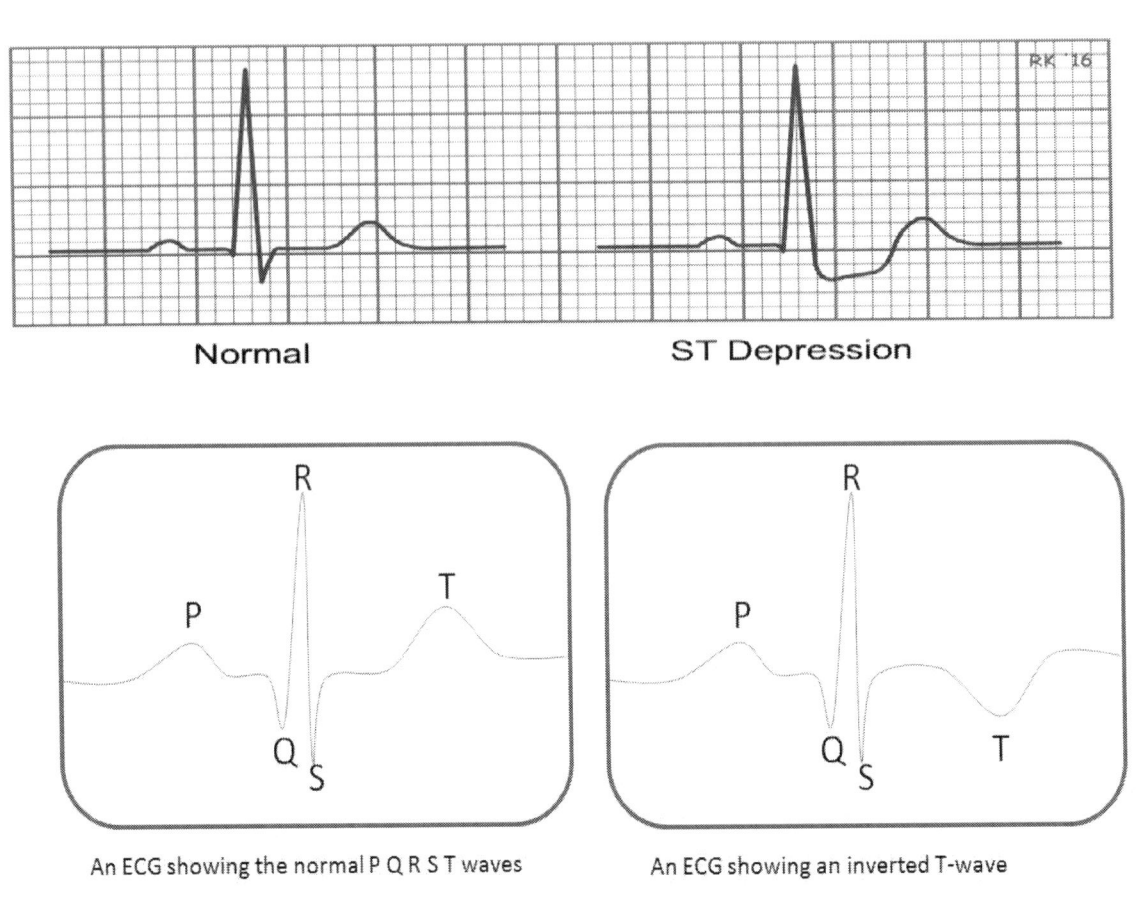

Normal | ST Depression

An ECG showing the normal P Q R S T waves | An ECG showing an inverted T-wave

With permission: Hill, M.A. (2019). UNSW Embryology (19th ed.) Retrieved January 7, 2019, from https://embryology.med.unsw.edu.au

SUMMARY

ECG **Primary Survey** provides a simple clinical algorithm that identifies acute cardiac emergencies and prioritizes interventions based on the following four questions:

1. Is heart rate too fast or too slow causing cardiovascular instability?
2. Is rhythm supraventricular or ventricular?
3. Are ST segments consistent with STEMI / NSTEMI?
4. Are T waves consistent with STEMI / NSTEMI?

On-scene 12 lead ECG and first responders' recognition of cardiogenic shock secondary to abnormal heart rates, potentially fatal ventricular arrhythmias, and STEMI / NSTEMI affects patient morbidity and mortality. STEMI / NSTEMI alerts allow receiving institutions to ready catheterization laboratories for percutaneous coronary intervention. If hospital protocol permits, such patients may bypass over-crowded emergency departments on arrival and proceed directly to the catheterization suite. First responders' ability to perform ECG Primary Survey that identifies problematic heart rates, ventricular arrhythmias, STEMI and NSTEMI, represents a skill set that can expedite treatment strategies and improve patient outcomes.

INTRODUCTION: ECG PRIMARY SURVEY

Video Companion link: https://youtu.be/a-fx6Bgylrs

Timestamp 3:12

The following section contains 26 ECGs for review and practice. Perform a Primary Survey on each. A YouTube link at the bottom of each ECG provides a detailed explanation of the case as well as timestamp for easy location. To gain the most benefit from this exercise, view the video link only after completing your Primary Survey.

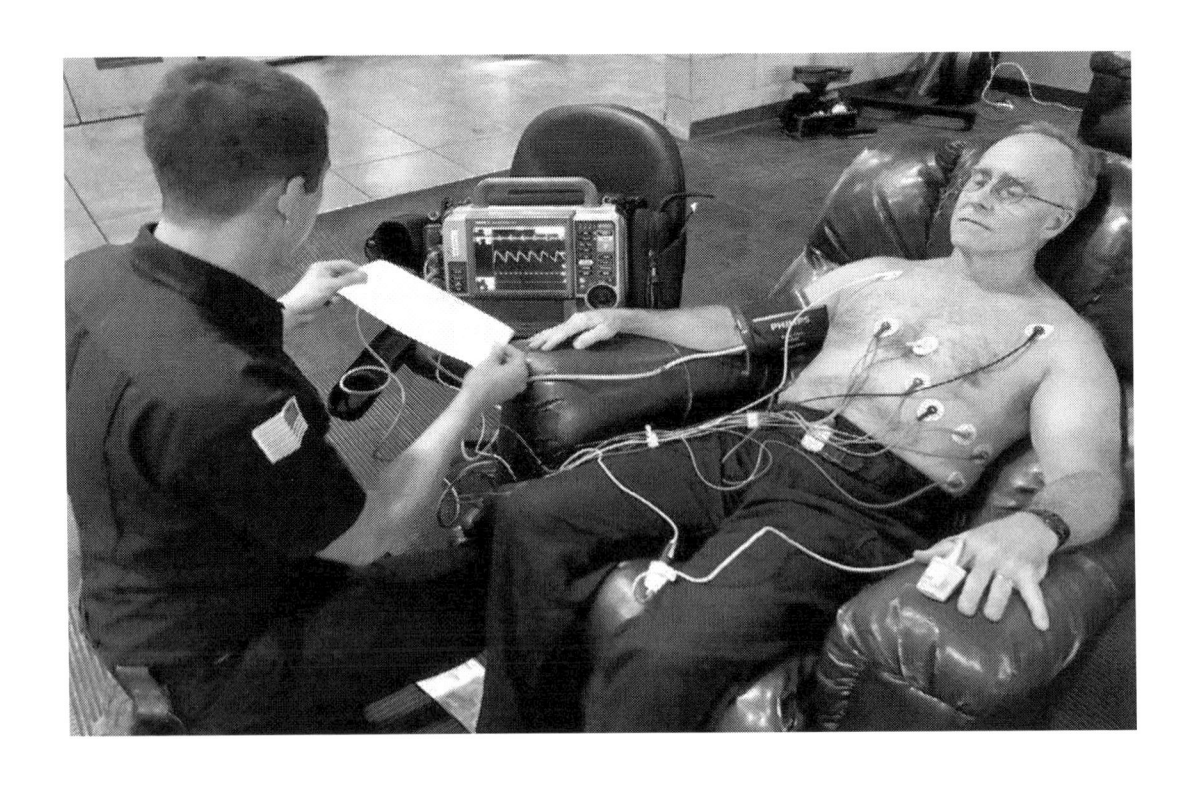

ECG FOR FIRST RESPONDERS
ECG CASES 3 - 26

The following ECGs taken from ECG Wave-Maven: Self-Assessment Program for Students and Clinicians. http://ecg.bidmc.harvard.edu do not display one mm square divisions. Each square represents five mm. In deciding whether a rhythm is ventricular in nature, assume ventricular if the QRS spans more than half the five mm square.

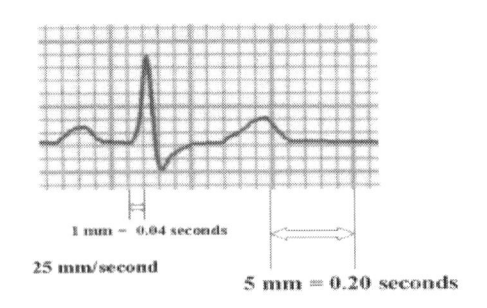

1 mm = 0.04 seconds
25 mm/second
5 mm = 0.20 seconds

Case 3: Forty-nine-year-old male complaining of chest pain. BP 146/88, respirations 16/minute. Temperature 99°F. On-scene 12 lead ECG below.

NOTE: EACH SQUARE REPRESENTS FIVE 1 MM SQUARES IN THE FOLLOWING ECGS

Primary Survey

Rate causing cardiovascular instability?
Rhythm? Supraventricular or Ventricular
ST Segments? Normal or Abnormal
T waves? Normal or Abnormal
STEMI Alert? Yes or No
NSTEMI Alert? Yes or No

This square represents FIVE 1 mm squares

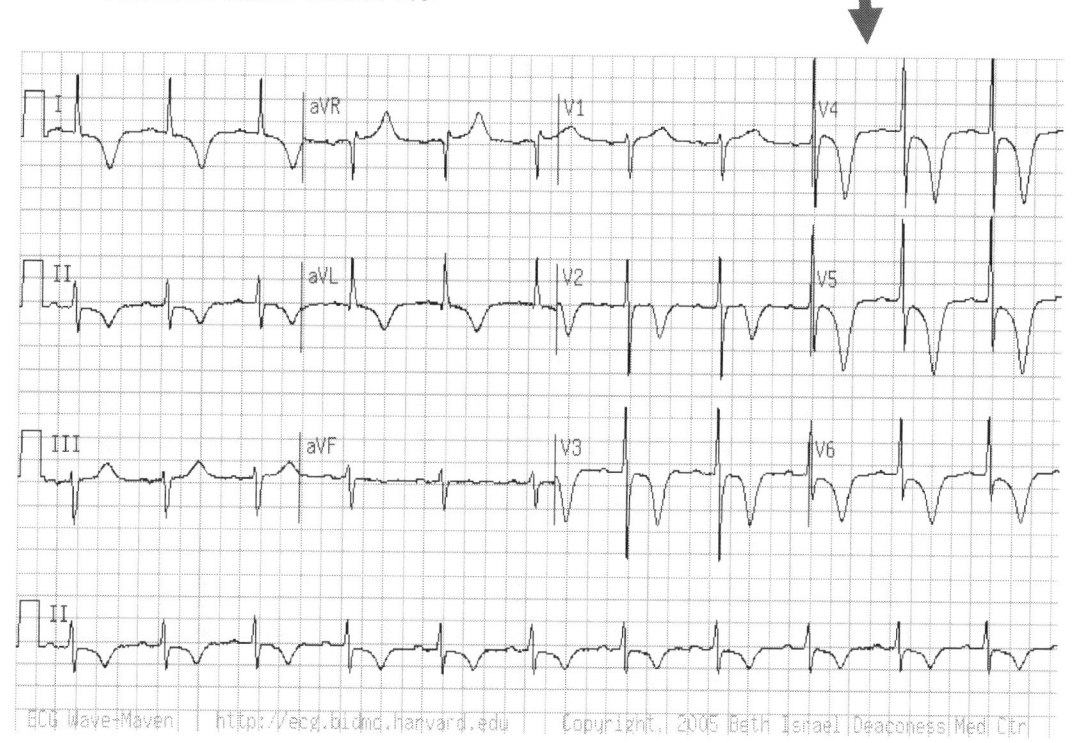

With Permission: Nathanson LA, McClennen S, Safran C, Goldberger AL. ECG Wave-Maven: Self-Assessment Program for Students and Clinicians. http://ecg.bidmc.harvard.edu.

Video Companion link: https://youtu.be/a-fx6Bgylrs

Timestamp 4:23

Case 4: Fifty-five-year-old schoolteacher complaining of nausea and substernal chest pain. Patient is diaphoretic, BP 160/98, respirations 14/minute. Temperature 98.8°F. On-scene 12 lead ECG below.

Primary Survey

Rate causing cardiovascular instability?
Rhythm? Supraventricular or Ventricular
ST Segments? Normal or Abnormal
T waves? Normal or Abnormal
STEMI Alert? Yes or No
NSTEMI Alert? Yes or No

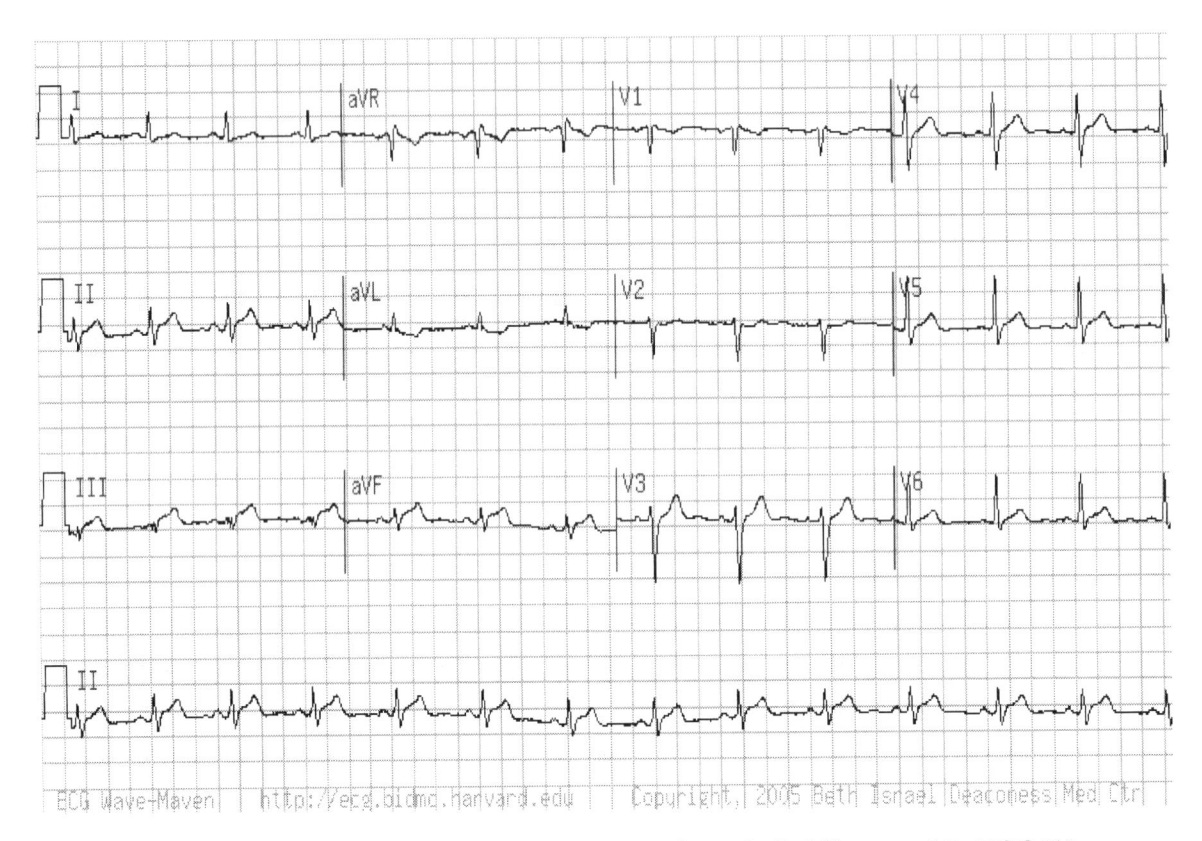

With permission: Nathanson LA, McClennen S, Safran C, Goldberger AL. ECG Wave-Maven: Self- Assessment Program for Students and Clinicians.
http://ecg.bidmc.harvard.edu.

Video Companion link: https://youtu.be/a-fx6Bgylrs

Timestamp 5:38

Case 5:
83-year-old widower with a history of advanced atherosclerotic cardiovascular disease complains of severe chest pain, BP 102/76, respirations 15/minute. Temperature 100°F. On-scene 12 lead ECG below.

Primary Survey

    Rate causing cardiovascular instability?
    Rhythm? Supraventricular or Ventricular ST
    Segments? Normal or Abnormal
    T waves? Normal or Abnormal
    STEMI Alert? Yes or No
    NSTEMI Alert? Yes or No

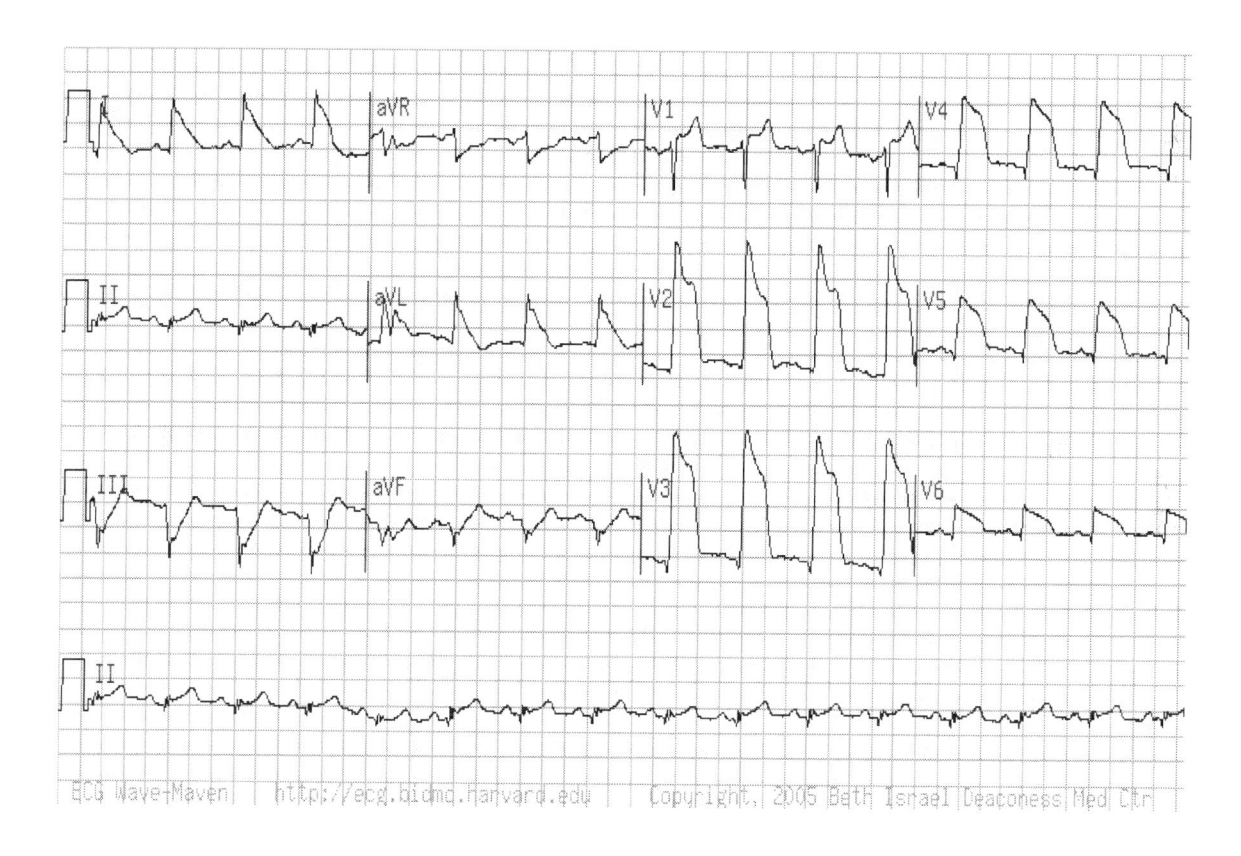

With permission: Nathanson LA, McClennen S, Safran C, Goldberger AL. ECG Wave-Maven: Self- Assessment Program for Students and Clinicians. http://ecg.bidmc.harvard.edu.

Video Companion link: https://youtu.be/a-fx6Bgylrs

Timestamp 7:03

Case 6: 54-year-old diabetic female with complaints of epigastric discomfort, nausea, and light-headedness, BP 124/82, respirations 16/minute. Temperature 98°F. On-scene 12 lead ECG below.

Primary Survey

Rate causing cardiovascular instability?
Rhythm? Supraventricular or Ventricular
ST Segments? Normal or Abnormal
T waves? Normal or Abnormal
STEMI Alert? Yes or No
NSTEMI Alert? Yes or No

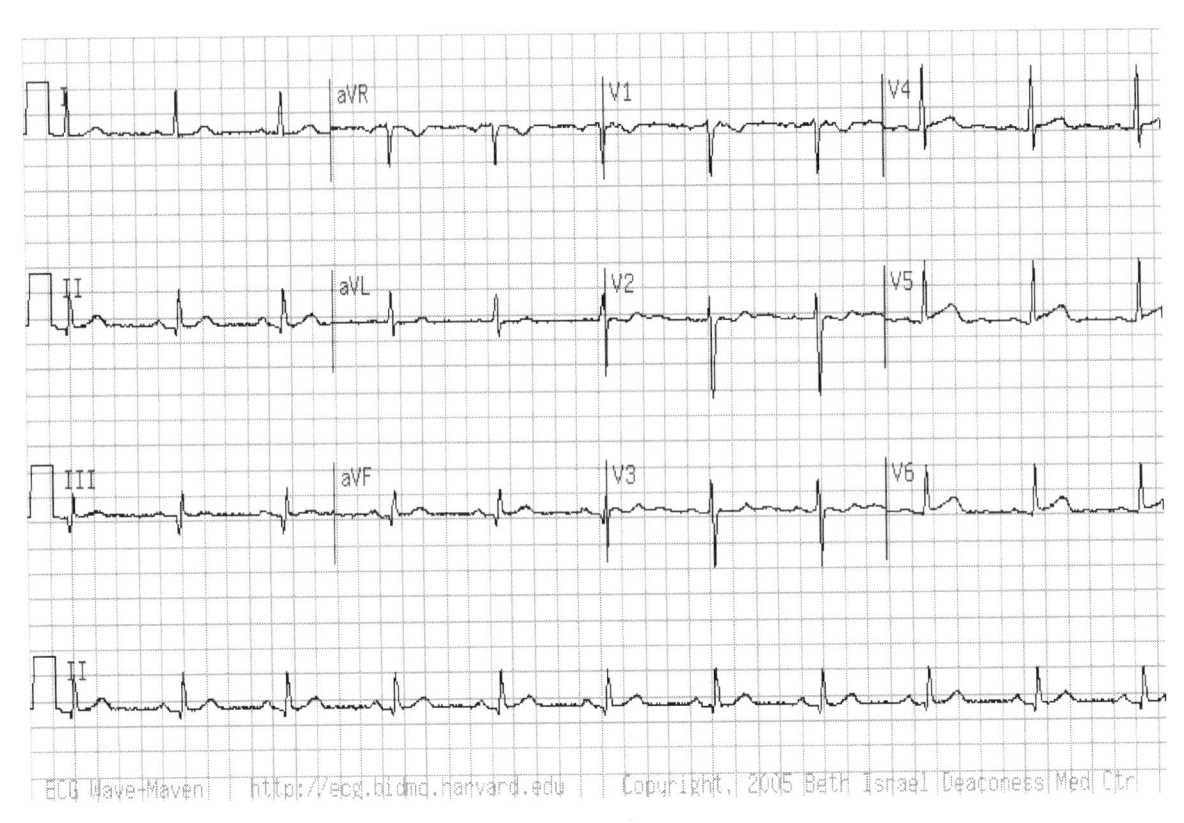

With permission: Nathanson LA, McClennen S, Safran C, Goldberger AL. ECG Wave-Maven: Self- Assessment Program for Students and Clinicians. http://ecg.bidmc.harvard.edu.

Video Companion link: https://youtu.be/a-fx6Bgylrs

Timestamp 8:41

Case 7: 44-year-old firefighter with substernal chest pain radiating to his left jaw, BP 152/90, respirations 14/minute. Temperature 99.2°F. On-scene 12 lead ECG below.

Primary Survey

Rate causing cardiovascular instability?
Rhythm? Supraventricular or Ventricular
ST Segments? Normal or Abnormal
T waves? Normal or Abnormal
STEMI Alert? Yes or No
NSTEMI Alert? Yes or No

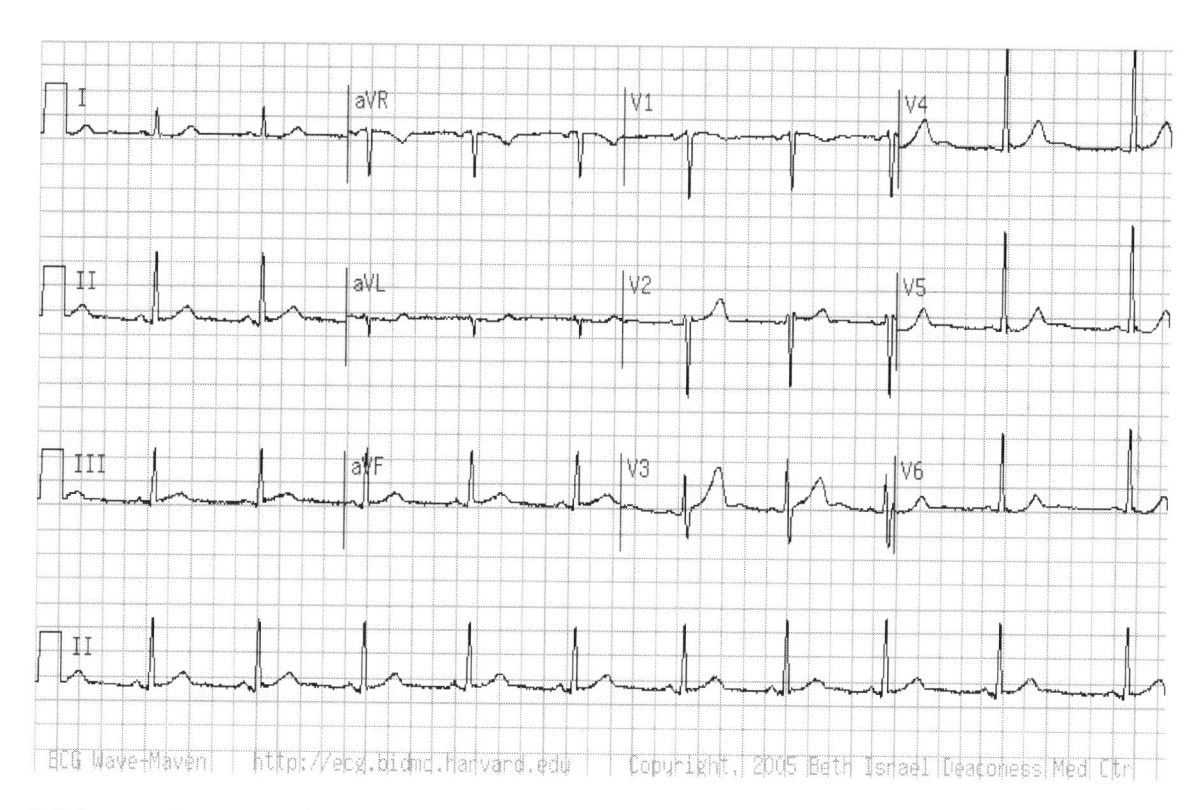

With permission: Nathanson LA, McClennen S, Safran C, Goldberger AL. ECG Wave-Maven: Self- Assessment Program for Students and Clinicians. http://ecg.bidmc.harvard.edu.

Video Companion link: https://youtu.be/a-fx6Bgylrs

Timestamp 9:58

Case 8: 63-year-old grandmother with squeezing chest pain, BP 106/70, respirations 18/minute. Temperature 99.4°F. On-scene 12 lead ECG below.

Primary Survey

- Rate causing cardiovascular instability?
- Rhythm? Supraventricular or Ventricular
- ST Segments? Normal or Abnormal
- T waves? Normal or Abnormal
- STEMI Alert? Yes or No
- NSTEMI Alert? Yes or No

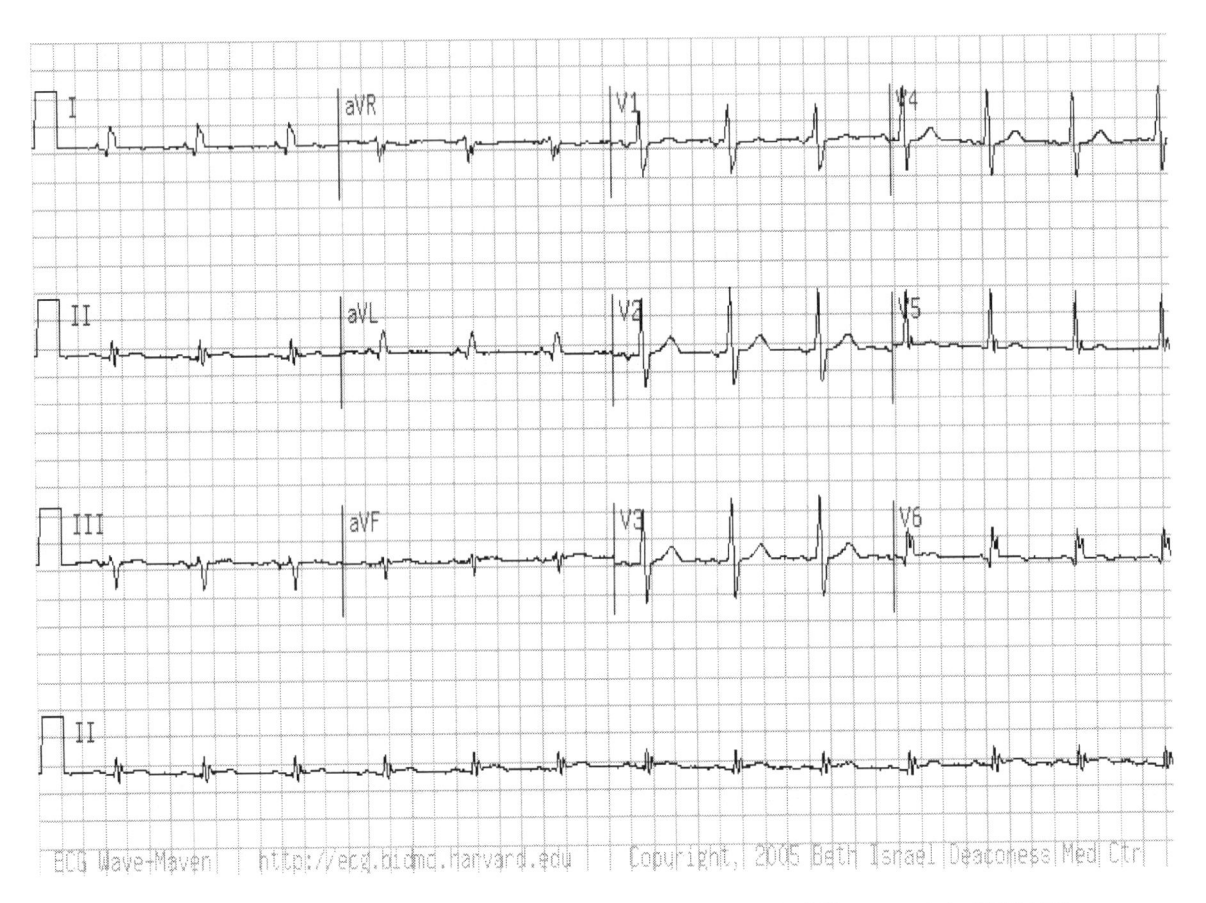

With permission: Nathanson LA, McClennen S, Safran C, Goldberger AL. ECG Wave-Maven: Self- Assessment Program for Students and Clinicians. http://ecg.bidmc.harvard.edu.

Video Companion link: *https://youtu.be/a-fx6Bgylrs*

Timestamp 11:03

Case 9: 76-year-old nursing home patient with complaints of weakness and shortness of breath, BP 112/76, respirations 13/minute. Temperature 100°F. On-scene 12 lead ECG below.

Primary Survey

Rate causing cardiovascular instability?
Rhythm? Supraventricular or Ventricular
ST Segments? Normal or Abnormal
T waves? Normal or Abnormal
STEMI Alert? Yes or No
NSTEMI Alert? Yes or No

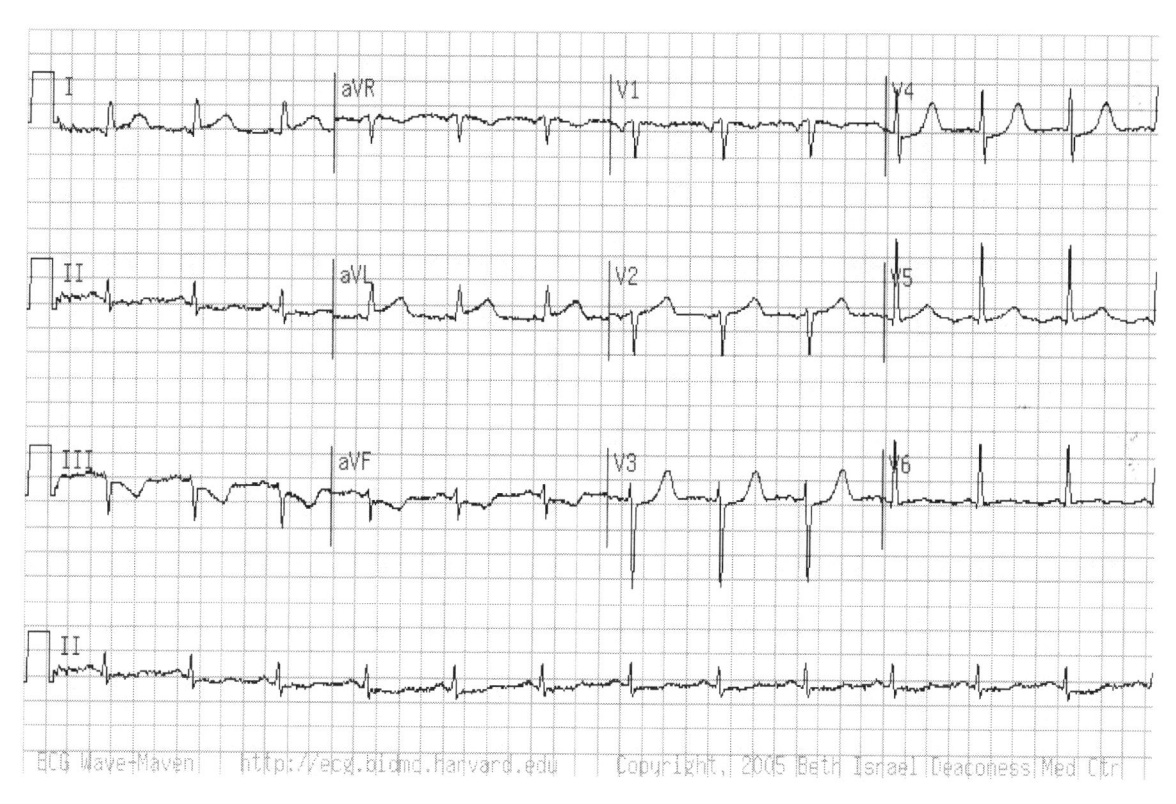

With permission: Nathanson LA, McClennen S, Safran C, Goldberger AL. ECG Wave-Maven: Self- Assessment Program for Students and Clinicians. http://ecg.bidmc.harvard.edu.

Video Companion link: https://youtu.be/a-fx6Bgylrs

Timestamp 12:42

Case 10: 48-year-old beautician complains of chest pain and shortness of breath. History of diabetes Type 2 and hypothyroidism, BP 138/86, respirations 18/minute. Temperature 98°F. On-scene 12 lead ECG below.

Primary Survey

Rate causing cardiovascular instability?
Rhythm? Supraventricular or Ventricular
ST Segments? Normal or Abnormal
T waves? Normal or Abnormal
STEMI Alert? Yes or No
NSTEMI Alert? Yes or No

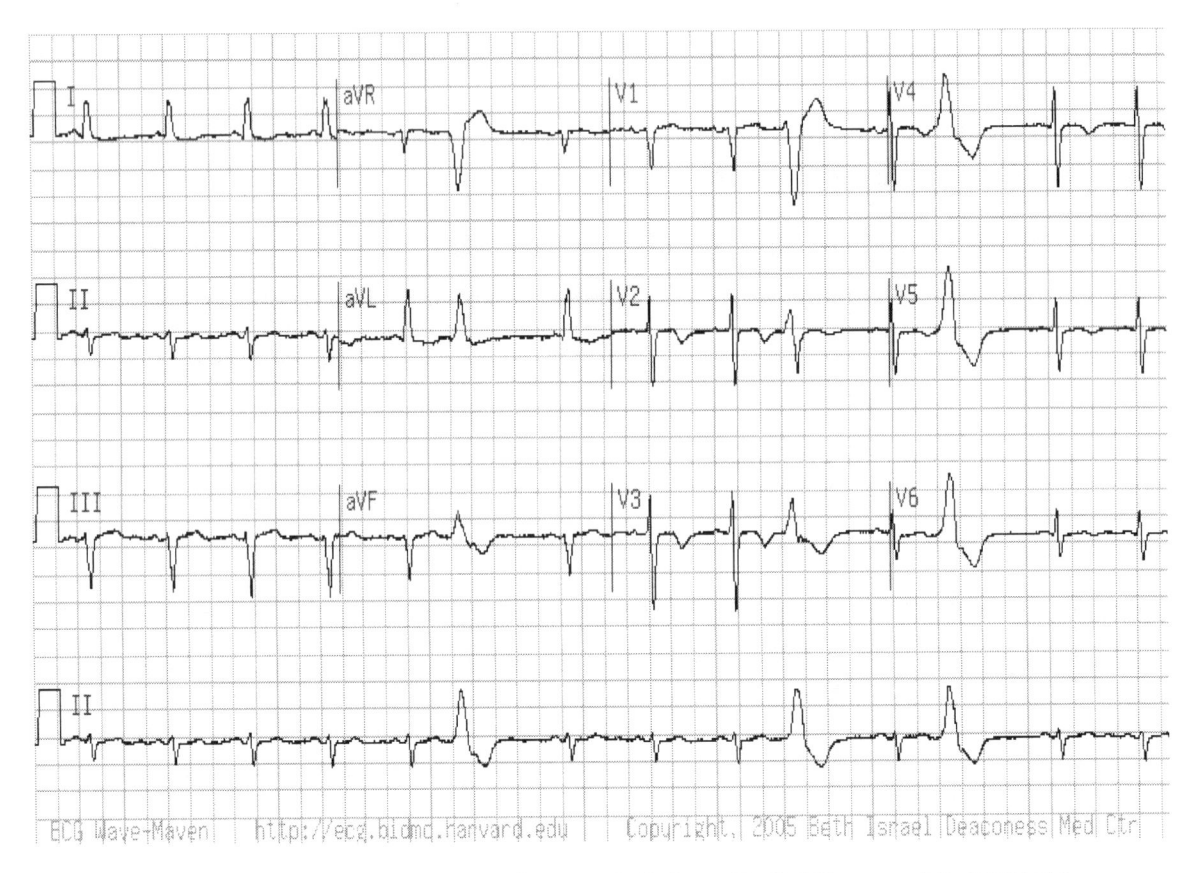

With permission: Nathanson LA, McClennen S, Safran C, Goldberger AL. ECG Wave-Maven: Self- Assessment Program for Students and Clinicians. http://ecg.bidmc.harvard.edu.

Video Companion link: https://youtu.be/a-fx6Bgylrs

Timestamp 13:52

Case 11:
33-year-old pipe fitter with complaints of palpitations for the past two hours. Heavy coffee drinker and 10-year pack history of cigarette smoking, Patient is sweaty and restless. BP 88/70, respirations 20/minute. Temperature 99°F. On-scene 12 lead ECG below.

Primary Survey

> Rate causing cardiovascular instability?
> Rhythm? Supraventricular or Ventricular
> ST Segments? Normal or Abnormal
> T waves? Normal or Abnormal
> STEMI Alert? Yes or No
> NSTEMI Alert? Yes or No

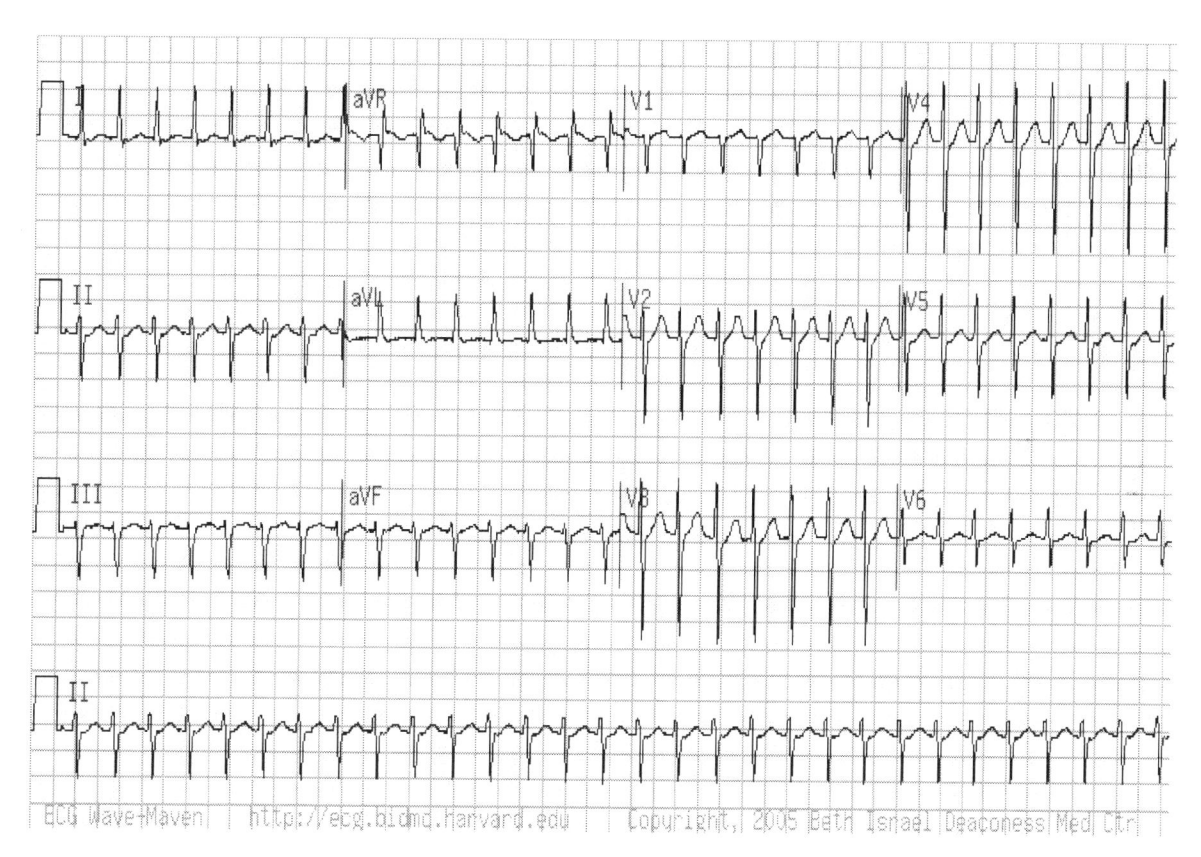

With permission: Nathanson LA, McClennen S, Safran C, Goldberger AL. ECG Wave-Maven: Self- Assessment Program for Students and Clinicians. http://ecg.bidmc.harvard.edu.

Video Companion link: https://youtu.be/a-fx6Bgylrs

Timestamp 15:46

Case 12: 58-year-old schoolteacher complains of chest pain radiating to her left arm, BP 158/94. Respirations 14/minute. Temperature 99°F. On-scene 12 lead ECG below.

Primary Survey

Rate causing cardiovascular instability?
Rhythm? Supraventricular or
Ventricular ST Segments? Normal or
Abnormal
T waves? Normal or Abnormal
STEMI Alert? Yes or No
NSTEMI Alert? Yes or No

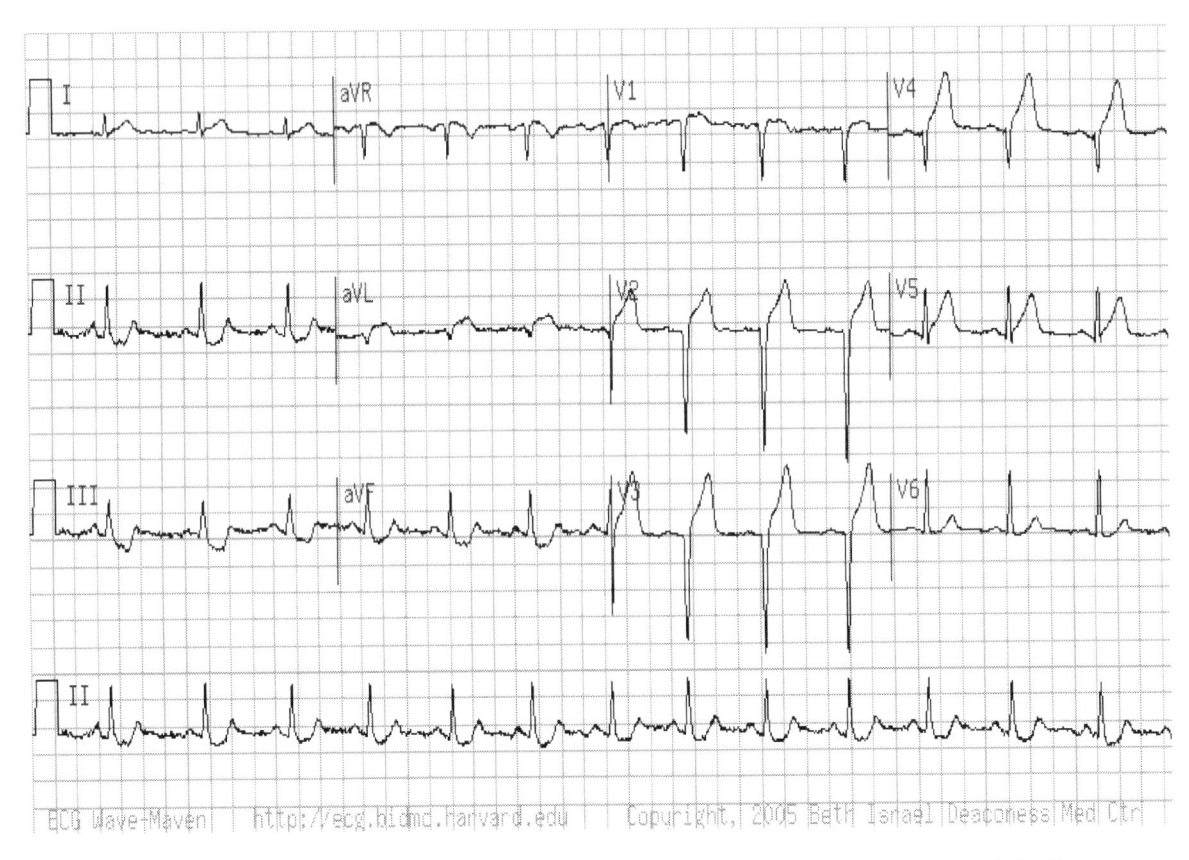

With permission: Nathanson LA, McClennen S, Safran C, Goldberger AL. ECG Wave-Maven: Self- Assessment Program for Students and Clinicians. http://ecg.bidmc.harvard.edu.

Video Companion link: https://youtu.be/a-fx6Bgylrs

Timestamp 17:35

Case 13: 44-year-old runner with complaints of cough for three weeks. Vital signs BP 110/70, respirations 14, Temperature 99°F. On-scene 12 lead ECG below.

Primary Survey

Rate causing cardiovascular instability?
Rhythm? Supraventricular or Ventricular
ST Segments? Normal or Abnormal
T waves? Normal or Abnormal
STEMI Alert? Yes or No
NSTEMI Alert? Yes or No

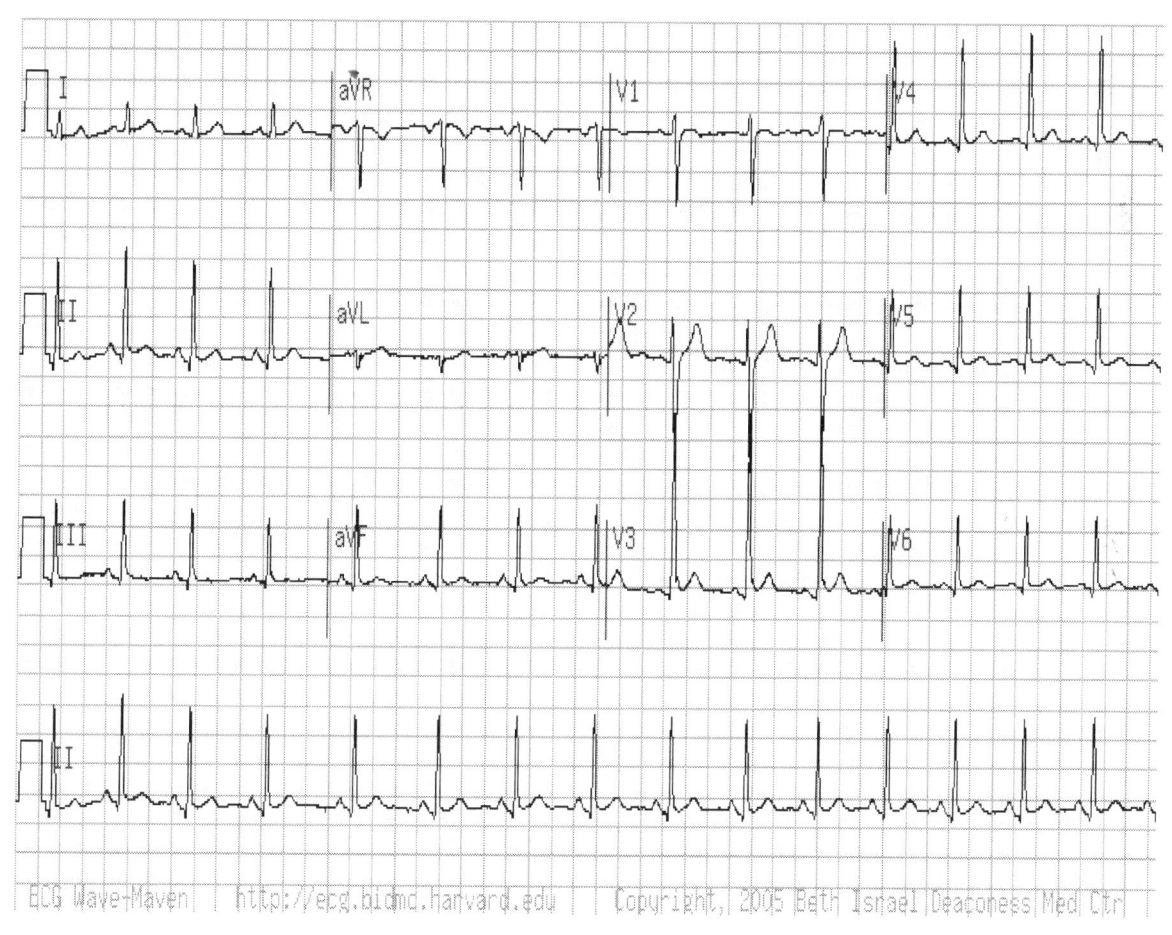

With permission: Nathanson LA, McClennen S, Safran C, Goldberger AL. ECG Wave-Maven: Self- Assessment Program for Students and Clinicians. http://ecg.bidmc.harvard.edu.

Video Companion link: https://youtu.be/a-fx6Bgylrs

Timestamp 18:40

Case 14: 70-year-old male in ICU post-resuscitation. BP 170/100, respirations 16/min. Temperature 99°F. On-scene 12 lead ECG below.

Primary Survey

Rate causing cardiovascular instability?

Rhythm? Supraventricular or Ventricular

ST Segments? Normal or Abnormal

T waves? Normal or Abnormal

STEMI Alert? Yes or No

NSTEMI Alert? Yes or No

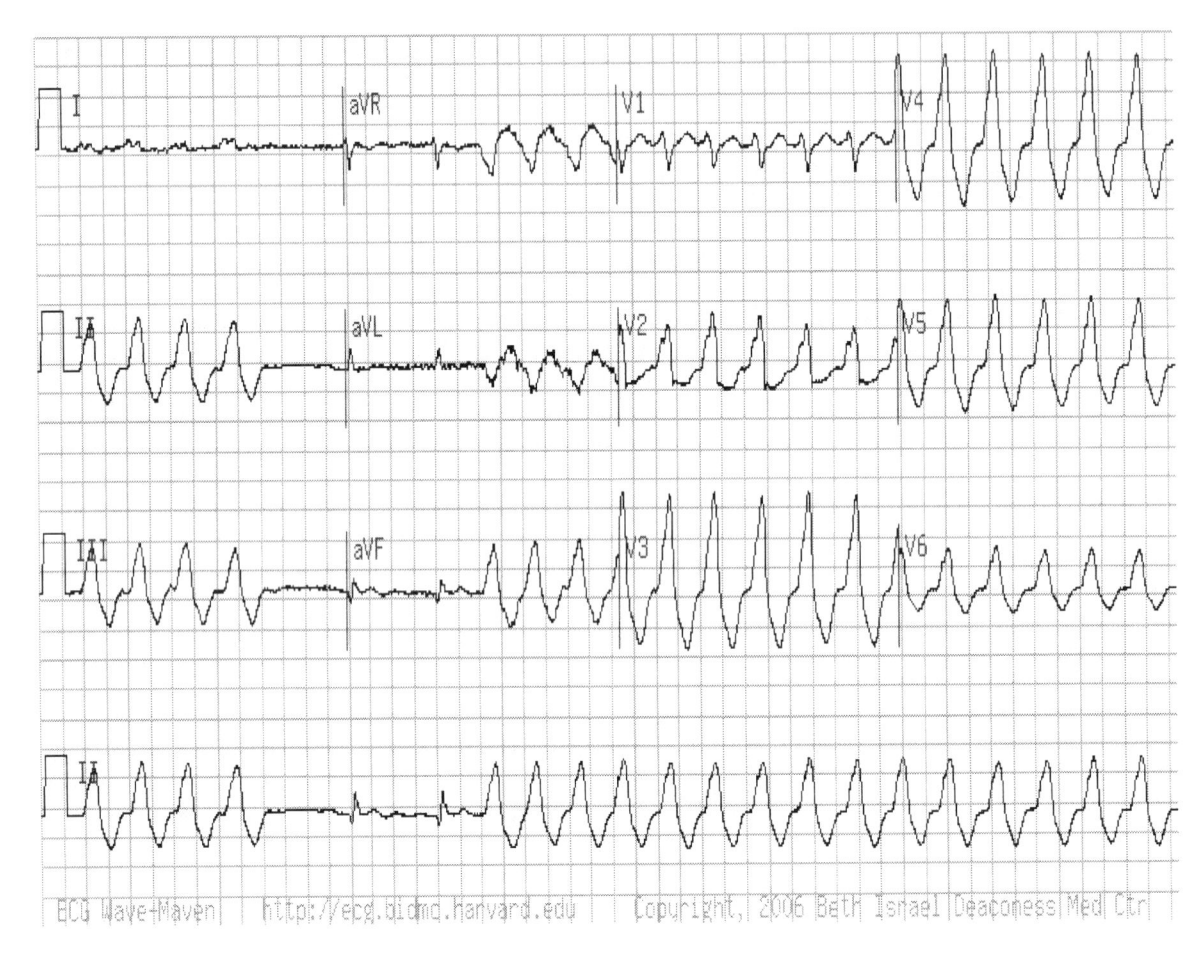

With permission: Nathanson LA, McClennen S, Safran C, Goldberger AL. ECG Wave-Maven: Self- Assessment Program for Students and Clinicians. http://ecg.bidmc.harvard.edu.

Video Companion link: https://youtu.be/a-fx6Bgylrs

Timestamp 20:43

Case 15: 30-year-old male with palpitations, BP 128/82. Temperature 98.2ºF. On- scene 12 lead ECG below.

Primary Survey

Rate causing cardiovascular instability?

Rhythm? Supraventricular or Ventricular ST
Segments? Normal or Abnormal
T waves? Normal or Abnormal
STEMI Alert? Yes or No
NSTEMI Alert? Yes or No

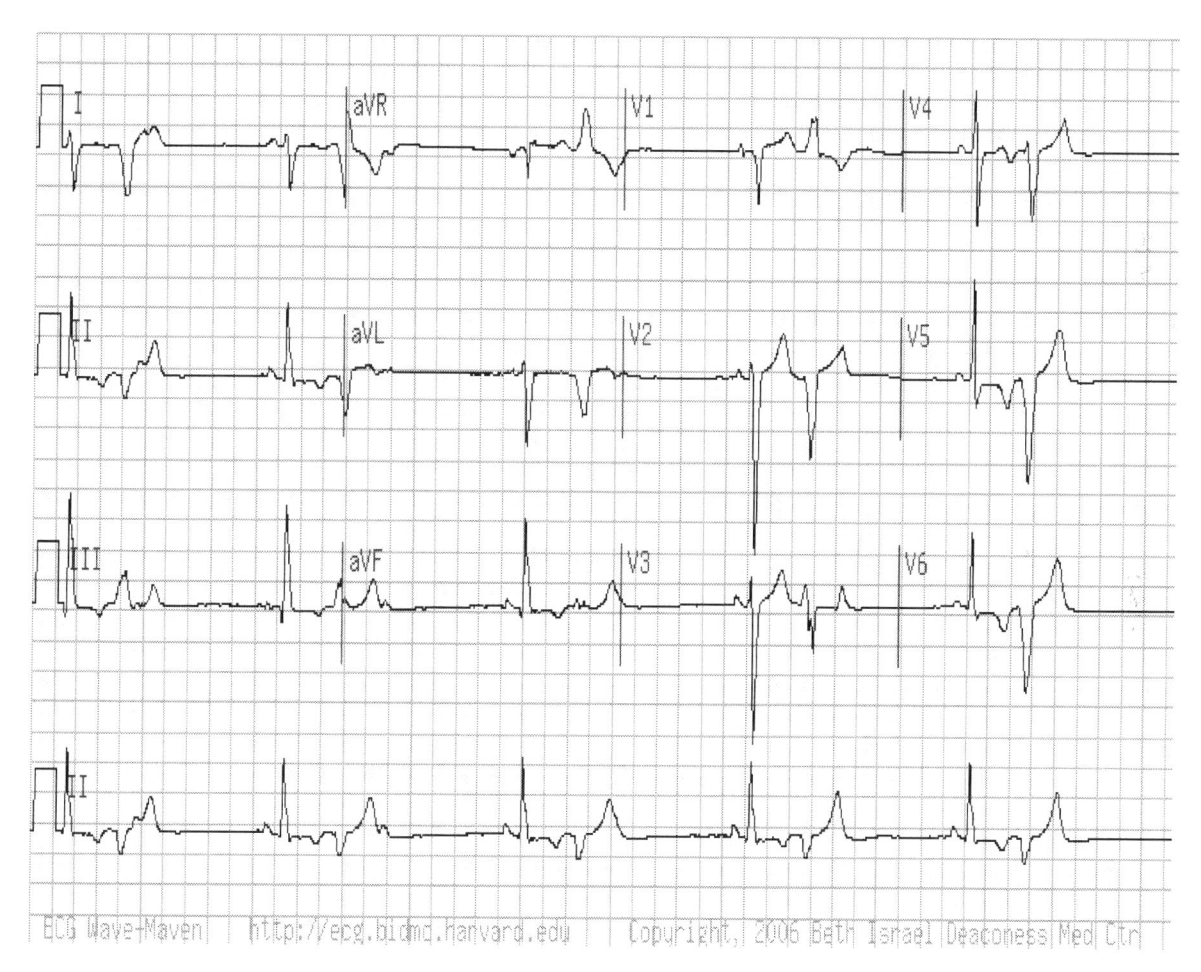

With permission: Nathanson LA, McClennen S, Safran C, Goldberger AL. ECG Wave-Maven: Self- Assessment Program for Students and Clinicians. http://ecg.bidmc.harvard.edu.

Video Companion link: https://youtu.be/a-fx6Bgylrs

Timestamp 22:04

Case 16: Elderly male, awake and alert, with weakness and indigestion, BP 166/94. Temperature 100.2°F. On-scene 12 lead ECG below.

Primary Survey

Rate causing cardiovascular instability?

Rhythm? Supraventricular or Ventricular

ST Segments? Normal or Abnormal

T waves? Normal or Abnormal

STEMI Alert? Yes or No

NSTEMI Alert? Yes or No

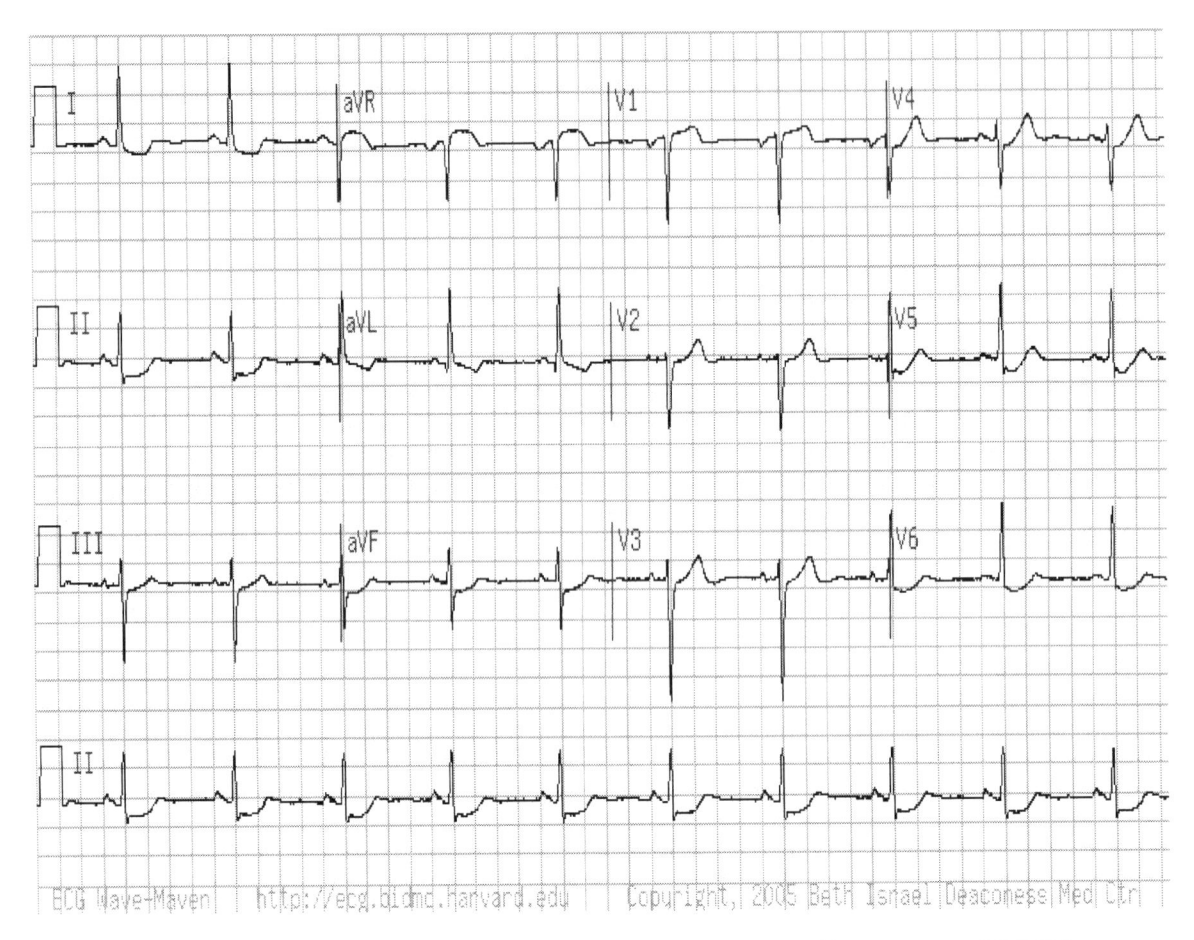

With permission: Nathanson LA, McClennen S, Safran C, Goldberger AL. ECG Wave-Maven: Self- Assessment Program for Students and Clinicians. http://ecg.bidmc.harvard.edu.

Video Companion link: *https://youtu.be/a-fx6Bgylrs*

Timestamp 23:57

Case 17: 66-year-old patient with history of Parkinsonism complains of sharp chest pain, BP 140/82. Respirations 18/minute. Temperature 98.6°F. On-scene 12 lead ECG below.

Primary Survey

Rate causing cardiovascular instability?
Rhythm? Supraventricular or Ventricular
ST Segments? Normal or Abnormal
T waves? Normal or Abnormal
STEMI Alert? Yes or No
NSTEMI Alert? Yes or No

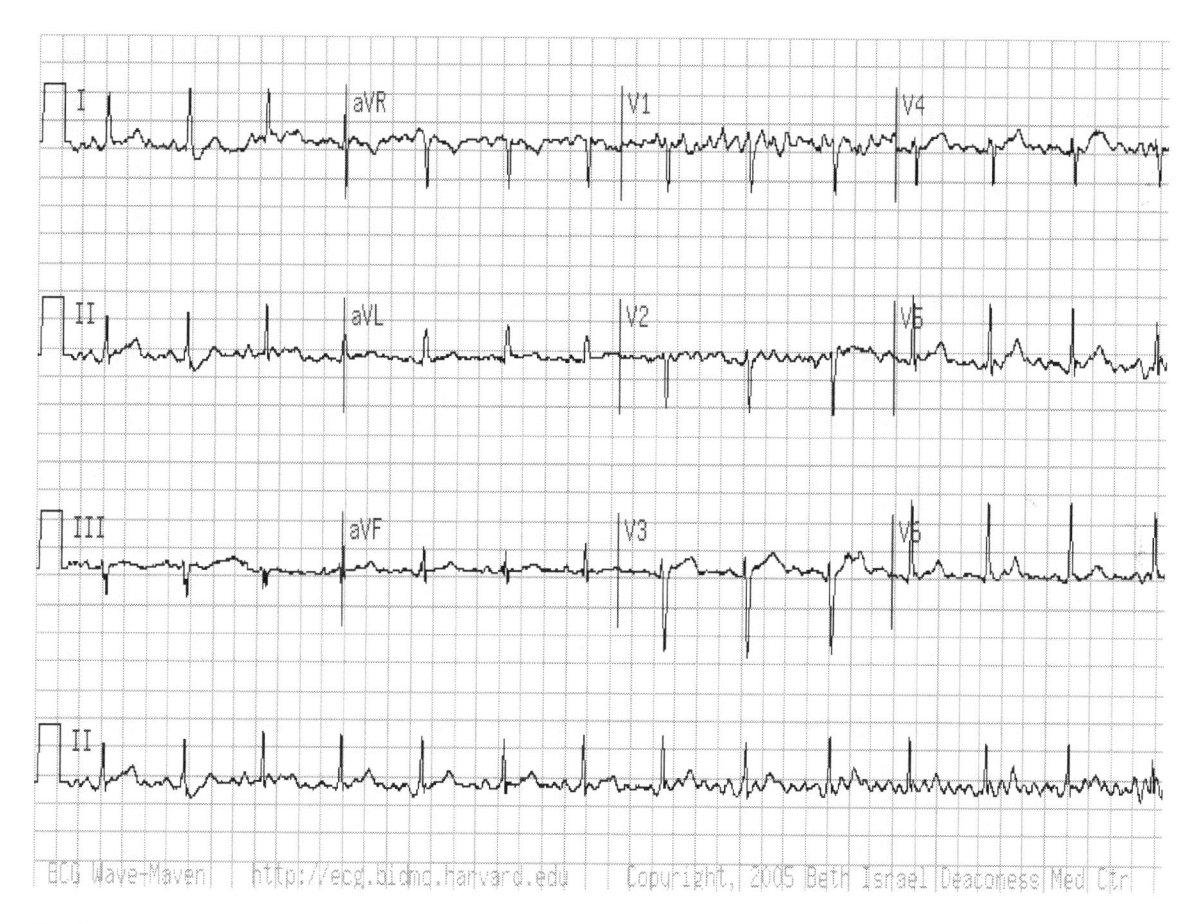

With permission: Nathanson LA, McClennen S, Safran C, Goldberger AL. ECG Wave-Maven: Self- Assessment Program for Students and Clinicians. http://ecg.bidmc.harvard.edu.

Video Companion link: https://youtu.be/a-fx6Bgylrs

Timestamp 25:06

Case 18
74-year-old retired sales executive with syncope and history of hypertension. Vitals BP 160/95, respirations 14/minute. Temperature 99.4°F. On-scene 12 lead ECG below.

Primary Survey

Rate causing cardiovascular instability?
Rhythm? Supraventricular or Ventricular
ST Segments? Normal or Abnormal
T waves? Normal or Abnormal
STEMI Alert? Yes or No
NSTEMI Alert? Yes or No

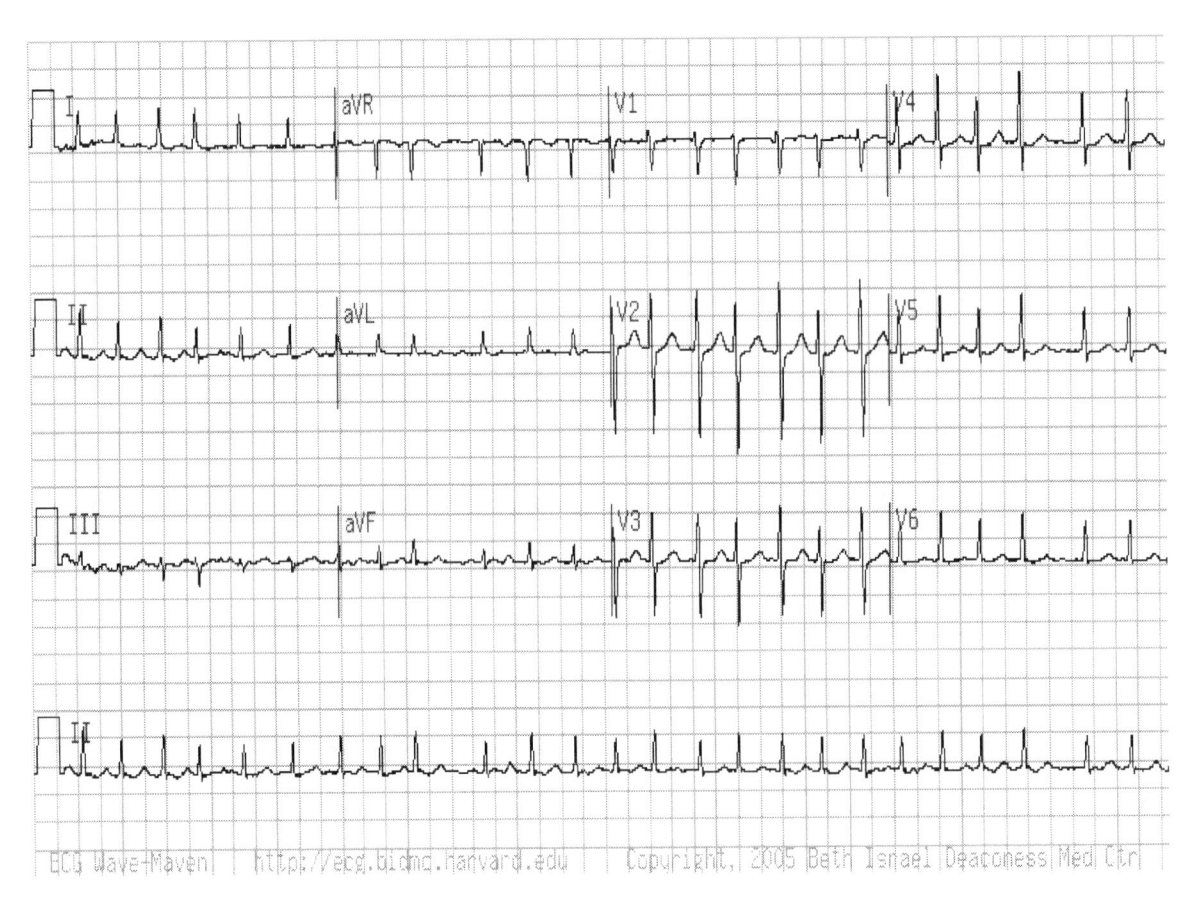

With permission: Nathanson LA, McClennen S, Safran C, Goldberger AL. ECG Wave-Maven: Self- Assessment Program for Students and Clinicians. http://ecg.bidmc.harvard.edu.

Video Companion link: https://youtu.be/a-fx6Bgylrs

Timestamp 26:46

Case 19: 31-year-old college student complaining of chest pain, BP 118/80, respirations 16/minute. Temperature 99°F. On-scene 12 lead ECG below.

Primary Survey

Rate causing cardiovascular instability?

Rhythm? Supraventricular or Ventricular ST
Segments? Normal or Abnormal
T waves? Normal or Abnormal
STEMI Alert? Yes or No
NSTEMI Alert? Yes or No

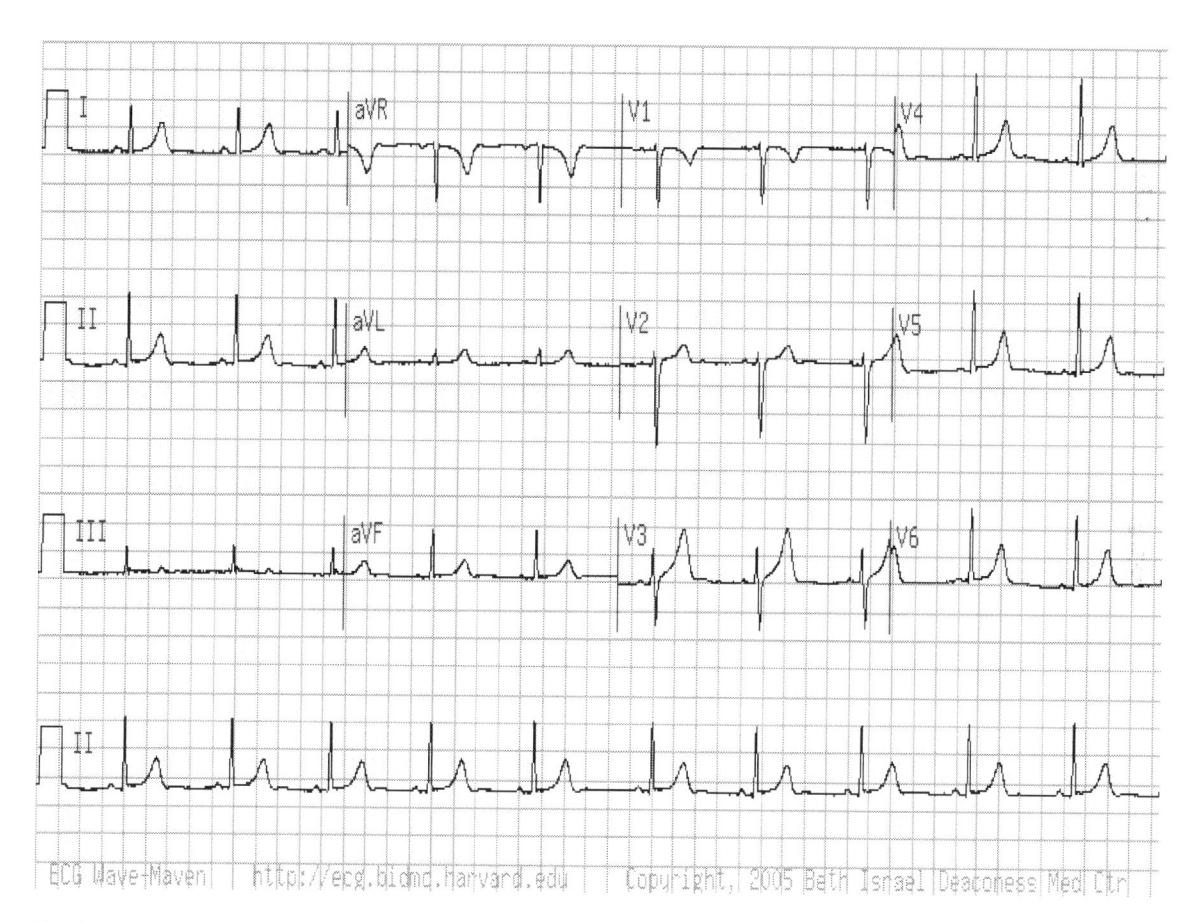

With permission: Nathanson LA, McClennen S, Safran C, Goldberger AL. ECG Wave-Maven: Self- Assessment Program for Students and Clinicians. http://ecg.bidmc.harvard.edu.

Video Companion link: https://youtu.be/a-fx6Bgylrs

Timestamp 28:42

Case 20: Middle-aged man found unconscious, BP -/- (unable to obtain). On-scene 12 lead ECG.

Primary Survey

    Rate causing cardiovascular instability?

    Rhythm? Supraventricular or Ventricular

    ST Segments? Normal or Abnormal
    T waves? Normal or Abnormal
    STEMI Alert? Yes or No
    NSTEMI Alert? Yes or No

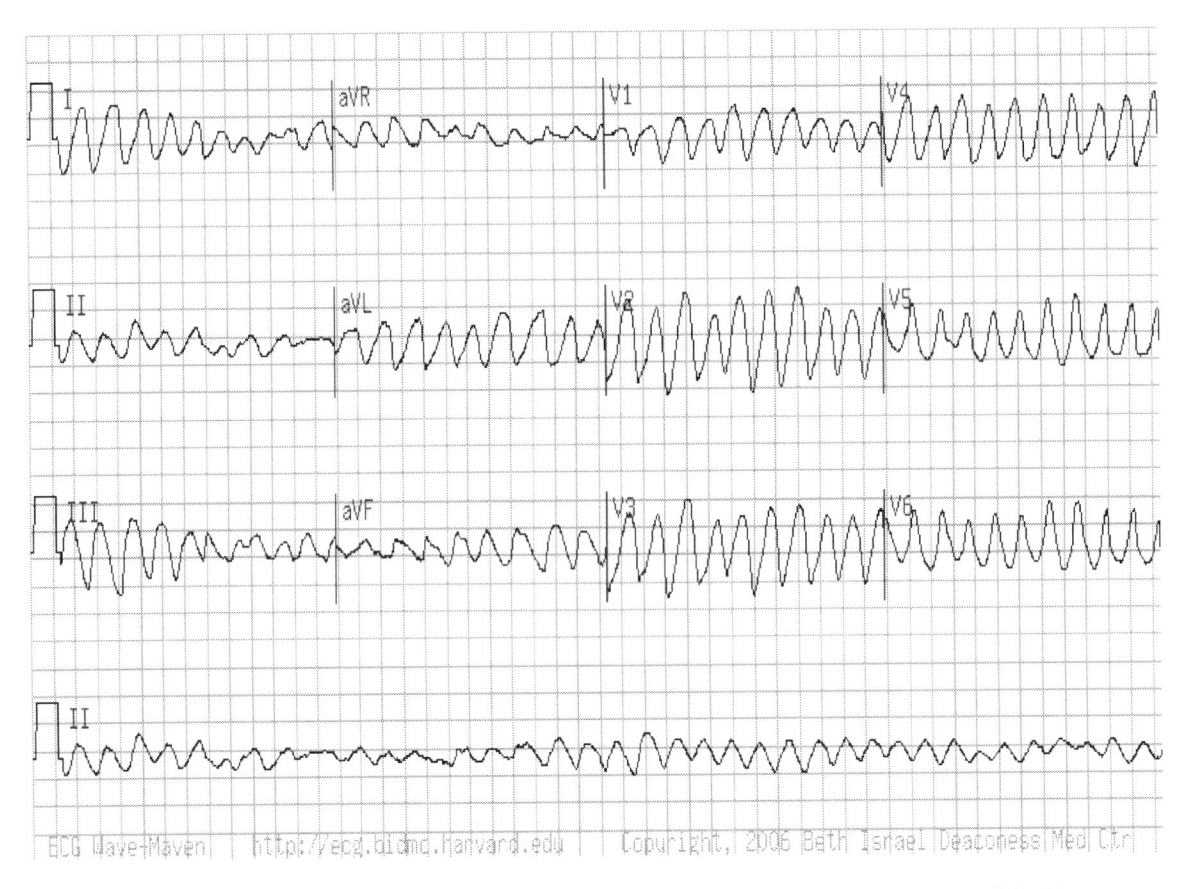

With permission: Nathanson LA, McClennen S, Safran C, Goldberger AL. ECG Wave-Maven: Self- Assessment Program for Students and Clinicians. http://ecg.bidmc.harvard.edu.

Video Companion link: https://youtu.be/a-fx6Bgylrs

Timestamp 29:42

Case 21: 51-year-old female with history of hypertension and diabetes complains of severe chest pain. BP 132/76, respirations 16/minute. Temperature 100.4°F. On-scene 12 lead ECG below.

Primary Survey

Rate causing cardiovascular instability?
Rhythm? Supraventricular or
Ventricular ST Segments? Normal or
Abnormal
T waves? Normal or Abnormal
STEMI Alert? Yes or No
NSTEMI Alert? Yes or No

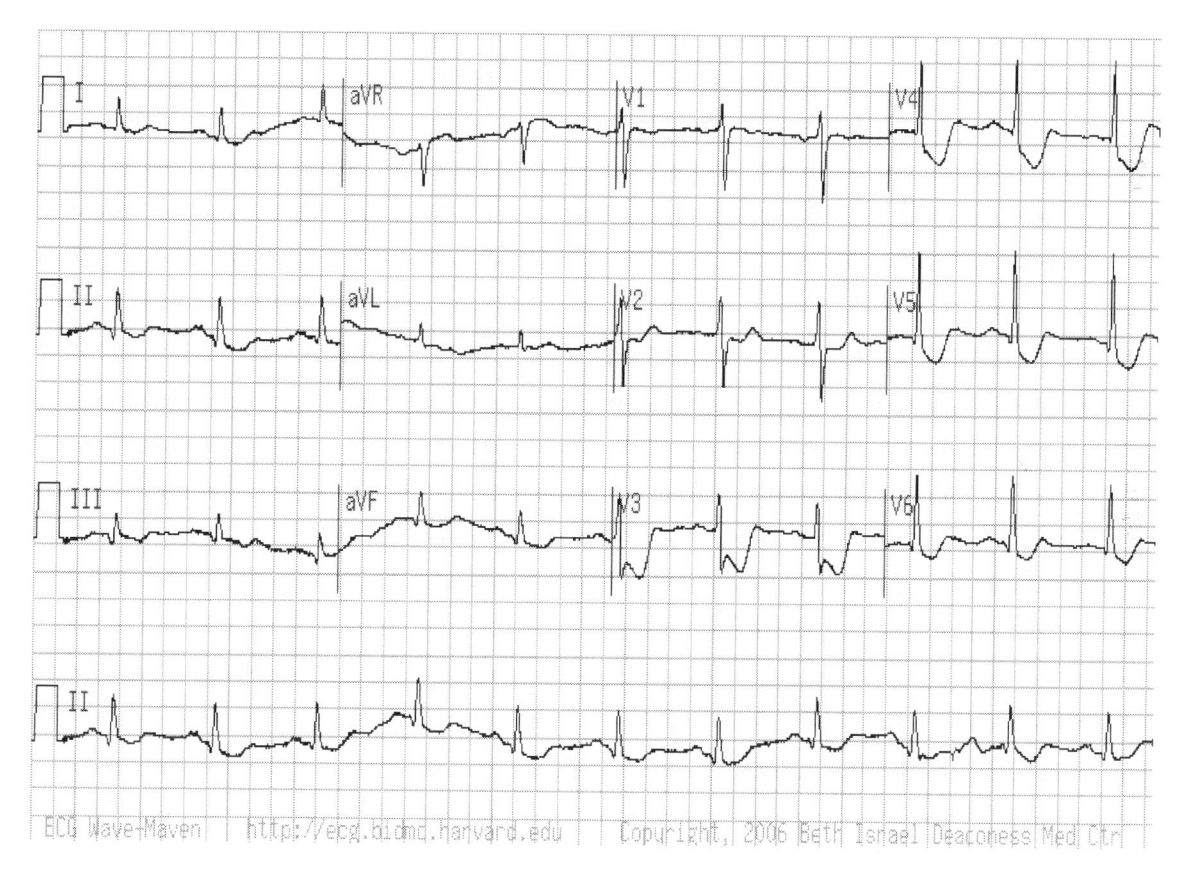

With permission: Nathanson LA, McClennen S, Safran C, Goldberger AL. ECG Wave-Maven: Self- Assessment Program for Students and Clinicians. http://ecg.bidmc.harvard.edu.

Video Companion link: https://youtu.be/a-fx6Bgylrs

Timestamp 30:43

Case 22: 18-year-old male complaining of chest pain at track meet. Vitals BP 125/80, respirations 16/minute. Temperature 98.8°F. On-scene 12 lead ECG below.

Primary Survey

    Rate causing cardiovascular instability?
    Rhythm? Supraventricular or Ventricular
    ST Segments? Normal or Abnormal
    T waves? Normal or Abnormal
    STEMI Alert? Yes or No
    NSTEMI Alert? Yes or No

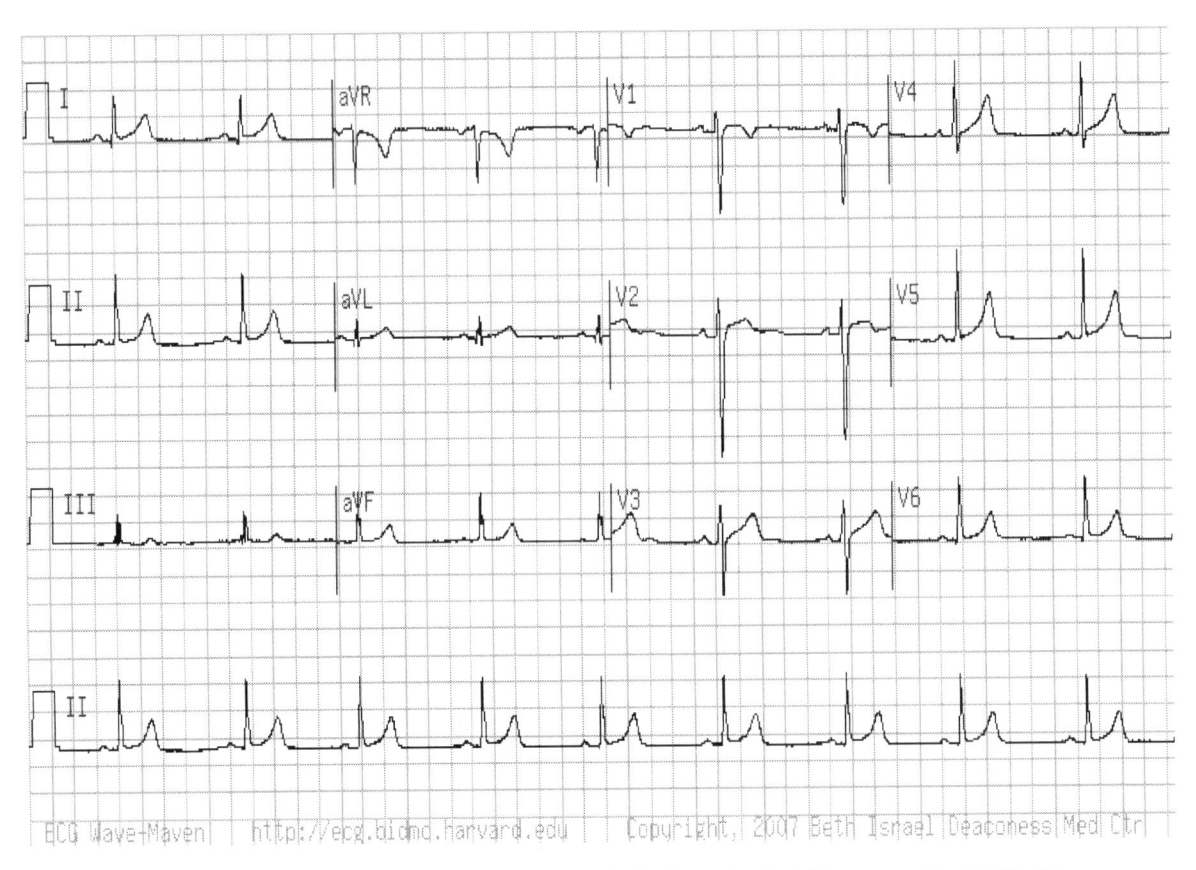

With permission: Nathanson LA, McClennen S, Safran C, Goldberger AL. ECG Wave-Maven: Self- Assessment Program for Students and Clinicians. http://ecg.bidmc.harvard.edu.

Video Companion link: https://youtu.be/a-fx6Bgylrs

Timestamp 31:48

Case 23: 66-year-old retired post office worker with complaints of shortness of breath and left-sided chest pain. BP 165/100, respirations 16/minute. Temperature 98.2°F. On-scene 12 lead ECG below.

Primary Survey

Rate causing cardiovascular instability?
Rhythm? Supraventricular or Ventricular
ST Segments? Normal or Abnormal
T waves? Normal or Abnormal
STEMI Alert? Yes or No
NSTEMI Alert? Yes or No

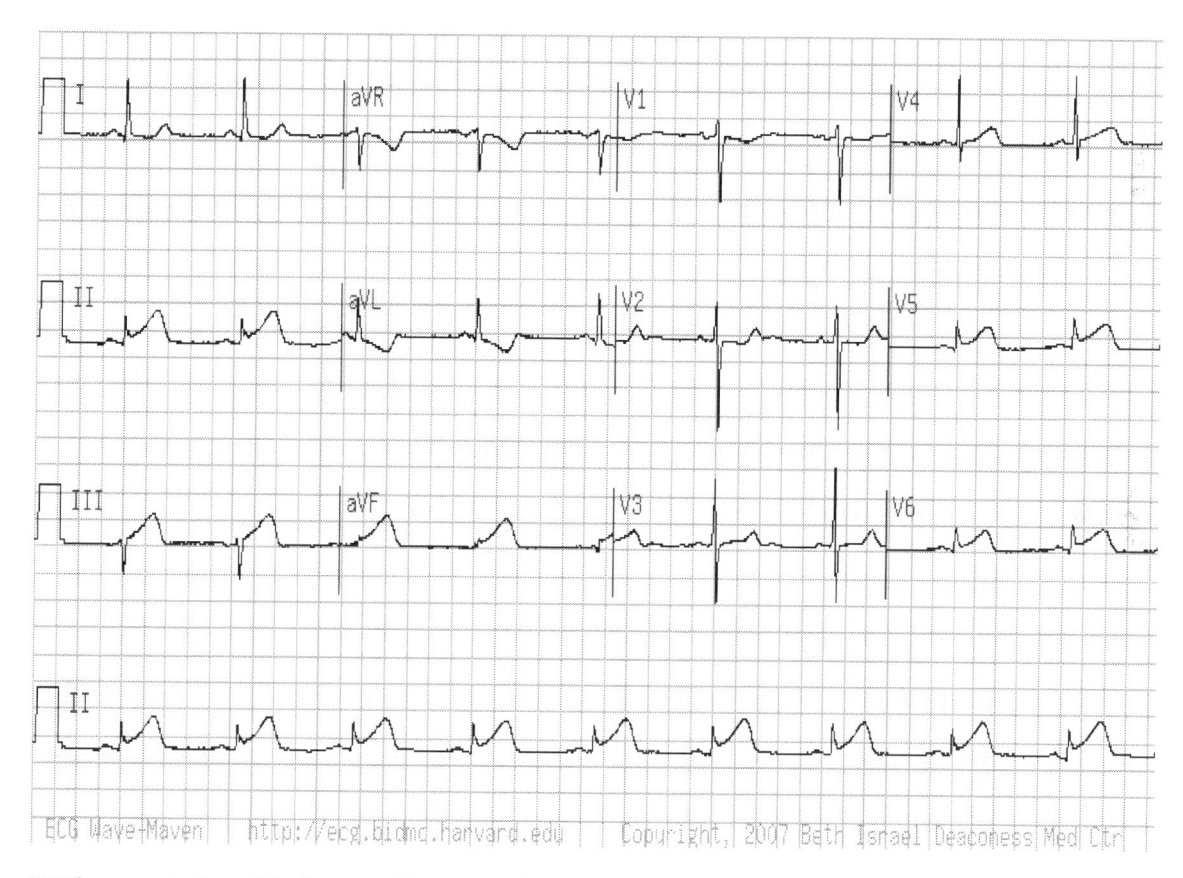

With permission: Nathanson LA, McClennen S, Safran C, Goldberger AL. ECG Wave-Maven: Self- Assessment Program for Students and Clinicians. http://ecg.bidmc.harvard.edu.

Video Companion link: https://youtu.be/a-fx6Bgylrs

Timestamp 33:47

Case 24: 49-year-old construction worker with acute chest pain, nausea, and vomiting, BP 130/84. Respirations 16/minute. Temperature 99.4⁰F. On-scene 12 lead ECG below.

Primary Survey

> Rate causing cardiovascular instability?
> Rhythm? Supraventricular or
> Ventricular ST Segments? Normal or
> Abnormal
> T waves? Normal or Abnormal
> STEMI Alert? Yes or No
> NSTEMI Alert? Yes or No

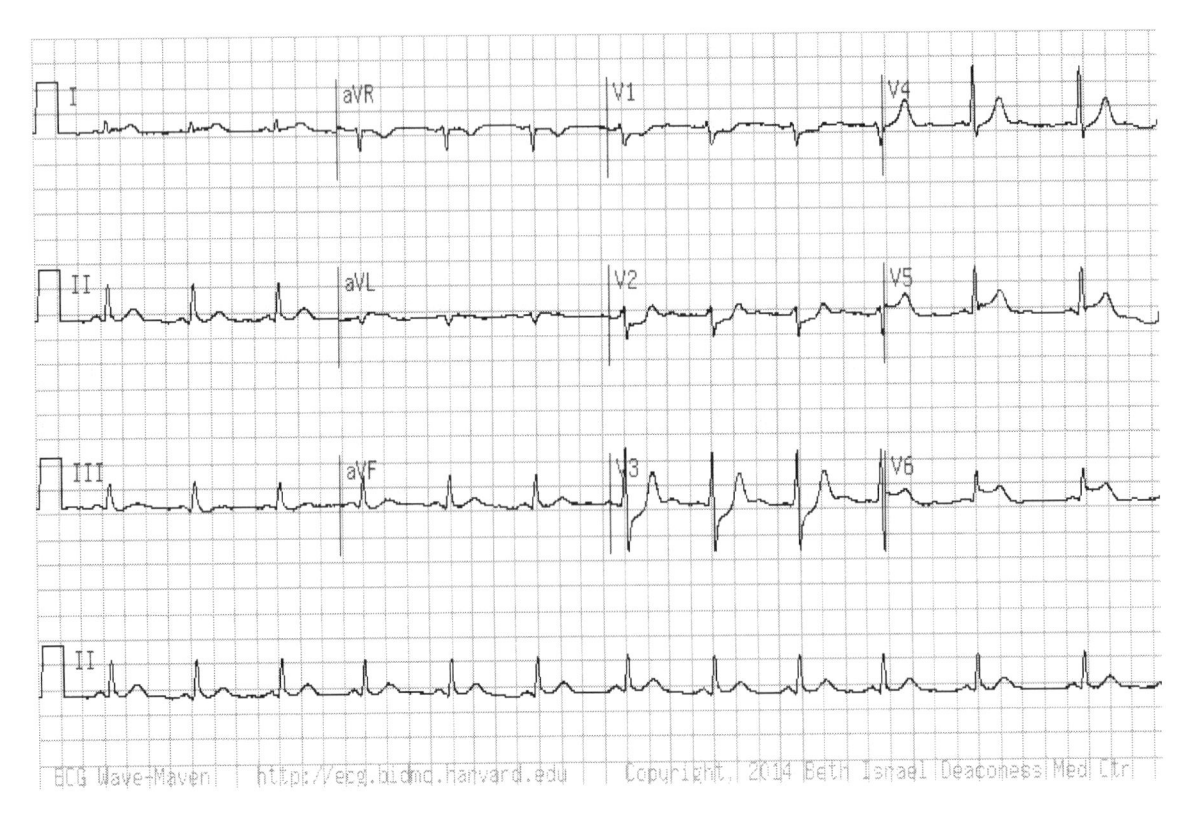

With permission: Nathanson LA, McClennen S, Safran C, Goldberger AL. ECG Wave-Maven: Self- Assessment Program for Students and Clinicians. http://ecg.bidmc.harvard.edu.

Video Companion link: https://youtu.be/a-fx6Bgylrs

Timestamp 35:12

Case 25: 33-year-old unrestrained male, MVA, with blunt chest trauma from steering wheel. Unconscious with BP 160/100, respirations shallow at 16s/minute. Temperature 99.6°F. On-scene 12 lead ECG below.

Primary Survey

    Rate causing cardiovascular instability?
    Rhythm? Supraventricular or Ventricular
    ST Segments? Normal or Abnormal
    T waves? Normal or Abnormal
    STEMI Alert? Yes or No
    NSTEMI Alert? Yes or No

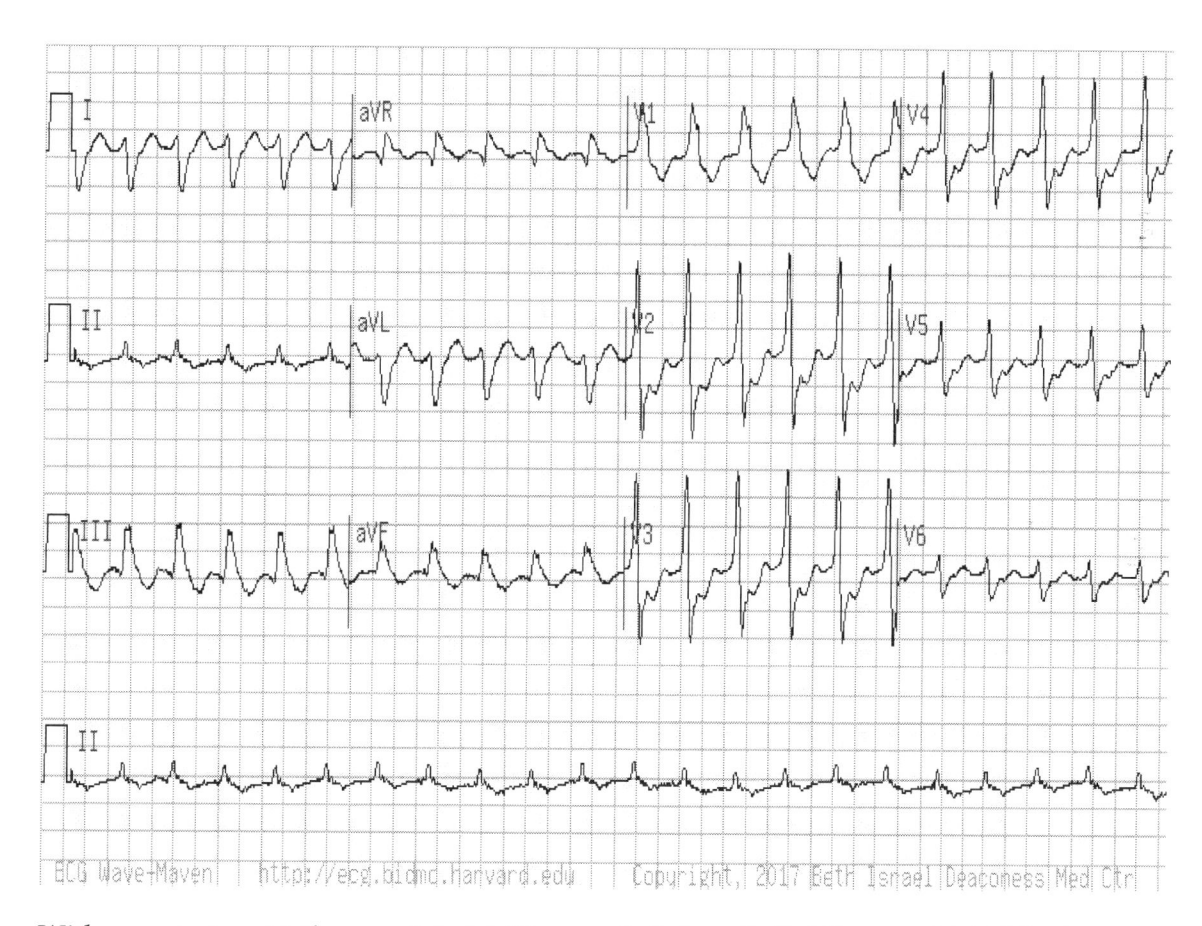

With permission: Nathanson LA, McClennen S, Safran C, Goldberger AL. ECG Wave-Maven: Self- Assessment Program for Students and Clinicians. http://ecg.bidmc.harvard.edu.

Video Companion link: https://youtu.be/a-fx6Bgylrs

Timestamp 36:10

Case 26: Thirty-eight-year-old mechanic complains of sharp pain on inspiration and non-productive cough. Medical history reveals a 10 year-pack/day cigarette smoking, BP 122/78. Respirations 18/minute. Temperature 100.2°F. Two ECGs performed on scene. Why?

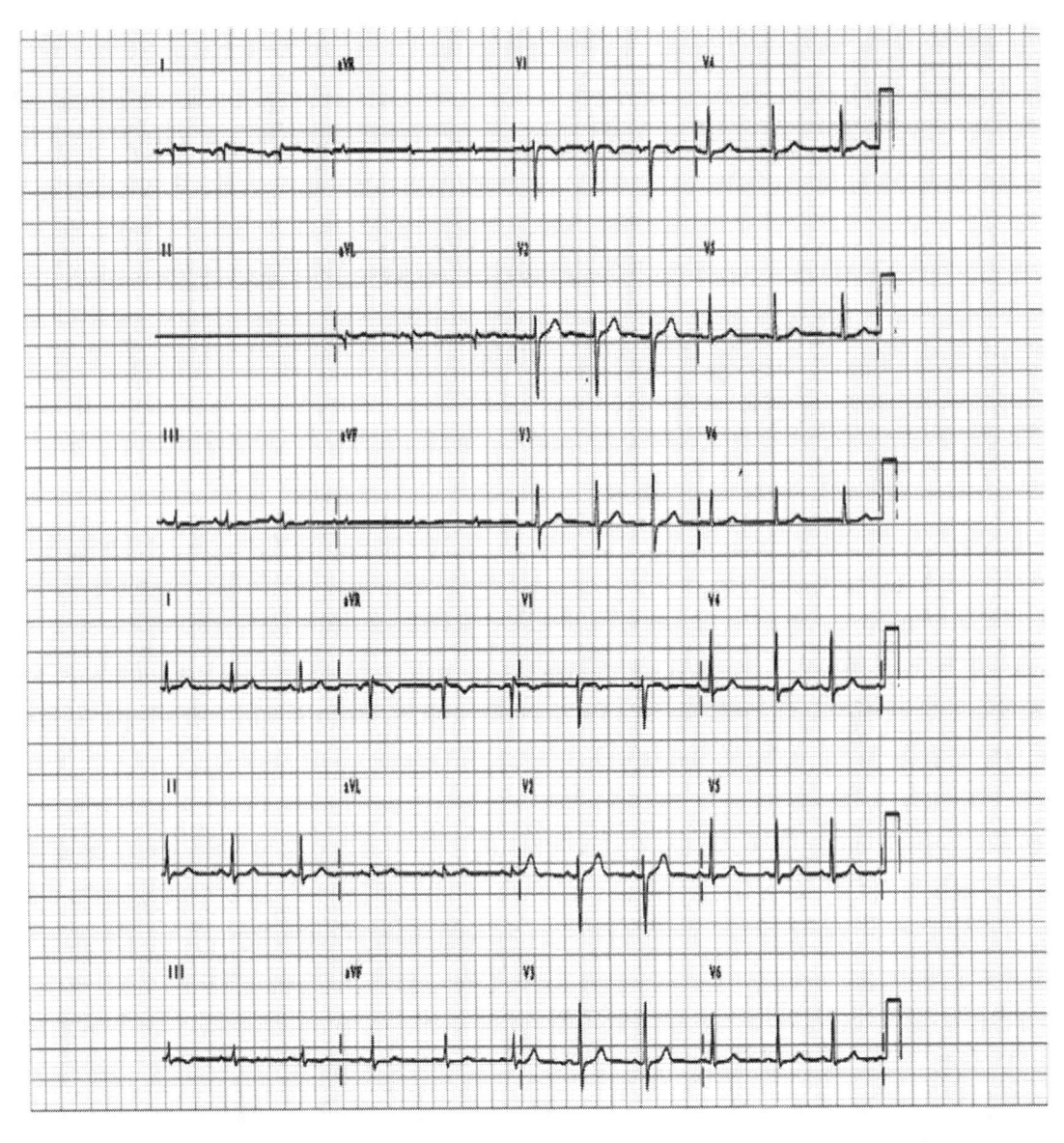

Video Companion link: https://youtu.be/a-fx6BgyIrs

Timestamp 37:28

SECONDARY SURVEY
TIMESTAMP 39:00
ADVANCED ECG FOR FIRST RESPONDERS

Printed in Great Britain
by Amazon